Sirtfood Diet:

a Science Based Guide

The Beginner's Guide for a Quick and Healthy Weight Loss.

Learn How Feeling Good Cooking 10 Super Easy Recipes that will Activate the Power of Skinny Gene.

Disclaimer

The information provided in this book is designed to provide helpful information on the subjects discussed. This book is not meant to be used, nor should it be used, to diagnose or treat any medical condition. For diagnosis or treatment of any medical problem, consult your own physician. The publisher and author are not responsible for any specific health or allergy needs that may require medical supervision and are not liable for any damages or negative consequences from any treatment, action, application or preparation, to any person reading or following the information in this book.

Table of Contents

Message for the Reader

Dear Reader,

I hope you can find interesting, inspiring and useful this book, "**Sirtfood Diet**".

Before you start this journey inside the world of Sirt Foods and the science behind them and their nutrients, take one minute of your time to consider the opportunity I am going to share with you.

The opportunity I am speaking about is the blog of my own, www.nutrifacta.com, at which you can subscribe freely.

Nutrifacta is the blog where I weekly publish articles dealing with food, science and wellness. If you are fond about scientific curiosities regarding food and how it interact with our body promoting health this is the blog that suits to you!

As the name says, Nutrifacta is about *Facts* of *Nutrition*, i.e. what is observable and verifiable (a fact). The content that I want to give weekly to Nutrifacta is therefore absolutely scientific, excluding what is not validated by scientific research. However, don't think of this blog as a boring scientific deep analysis full of abstruse terms of chemistry and physiology. Indeed, just alike I did in this book, I try to explain scientific content in a simple (but not simplistic) way, so that everyone can understand what I write without having studied biology or chemistry at school. In writing the articles for my blog I set myself the goal of being understandable even to a child but, at the same time, interesting for anyone who wants to improve the quality of his/her nutrition and his/her health through the knowledge present in the articles.

Therefore, consider the book you are going to read as the result of the same aim of my blog: telling the science behind food and the science behind the molecules that make up foods (the nutrients) trying to explain how they interact with our body and our biochemistry.

If, after reading this book, you will be satisfied with the scientific information I have given you and, above all, with the way I have given it to you, please consider to subscribe to Nutrifacta.com.

Why this book?

The world we live in puts an enormous strain on us to conform to an unhealthy lifestyle. Fast food outlets, eat-all-you-can offers, drive-through. The list has only started. The comfortable, fast-paced life we seek is inherently unhealthy and is the main reason so many of us are becoming overweight.

So, many people are looking in the wrong places to achieve optimal health and weight loss. Maybe you lose weight on a diet, but all too many leave you feeling tired, sluggish, give you headaches, acne, and require supplementary vitamins to see you through the day. They put a strain on your health when they should be improving it. And you are wondering if there are any healthy diets for weight loss or not.

Yes, you don't need to sacrifice your lifestyle completely, adjust its elements to make it a lot healthier.

Glad you pick this book!

When you are searching for diets for healthy weight loss, you might have two main reasons. Either you are overweight and want to find the best diet plan for weight loss, or you have already tried so many diets with very little or no results.

This and other reasons have always made me doubt in diets and in their effectiveness. In our common way of saying, being on a diet means being in deprivation, in a situation where food is removed from our tables and taste from our palate. I have always associated the word "diet" with something negative, unpleasant and as a source of painful sacrifices. I am sure that this feeling of mine is shared with many of us. Thus, I have always been "against" diets, simply because my professional career as a nutritionist and scientist has always warned me about diets. The science of nutrition (definitely one of the most fascinating sciences!) teaches us that the human body is a biochemical machine that needs a whole series of different molecules that it extracts from food to function. These molecules are named nutrients. It is essential that the supply of these nutrients is ensured constantly, otherwise our biochemical machine begins to no longer function at its best. Taking food off the tables often does not mean losing weight and improving your body composition. Maybe it does at the beginning, but in the long run the body begins to lose its efficiency and it can no longer perform all its functions effectively. Accumulation of excess weight and fat mass is one of the consequences that follows the absence of strength and energy to face the day.

We can roughly distinguish food into two categories: the "potentiating" foods, rich in nutrients useful to our body, on the one hand, and the "depotentiating" foods, low in nutrients, on the other hand. As you can see, I have not talked about low-calorie or high-calorie foods as, according to science, this takes second place. First of all, you need to give importance to foods rich in nutrients, this is the first goal to really feed us and eat to feel good and not just to fill our bellies. In general, high-calorie foods are the weakening ones (think of the junk food of fast food), but there are some exceptions, for example walnuts and dates, which are very caloric. However, as we will see, these foods, while providing many calories, also have a treasure trove of nutrients inside them and our body can only benefit from their intake.

My distrust of diets, however, was transformed after reading "The Sirt Food Diet", a book by Aidan Goggins and Glenn Matten that I invite you to read if you have not already done so. This book, in my opinion, has revolutionized the way we will all consider the word "diet" in the future to come. In fact, in the Sirtfood diet the imperative is not "to remove" but "to add": Sirtfood diet does not aim to remove calories (actually, it does only at the beginning of the diet for a very limited period of time) but to add nutrients! Sirtfood diet focuses on some specific foods and invites you to eat them in abundance (I dare to say until being full and satisfied with your meals!). These foods, named Sirt Foods, are all delicious and do not exclude other foods. Indeed the important thing is that Sirt Foods are present, then if we are particularly fond of another food not present in the list, we can associate it with Sirt Foods without any problem. This is very important because it allows a constancy of application that in a restrictive diet is not psychologically possible, if not at the cost of great sacrifices.

In other words, the Sirtfood Diet Plan lifestyle concentrates on maintaining a balanced diet and a good relationship between food and body at all times. You will be eating only food with a high nutritional value.

Forget the old-fashioned depressing diets! The promise of Sirtfood diet is to lose weight without starving yourself and even by consuming foods often prohibited in other diets!

Far From Being a Miracle Diet

According to the experts, the Sirtfood diet would even replace sports: the consumption of Sirt Foods would produce the same effect as a sports session in terms of eliminating fat, stimulating muscles, and even maintaining physical health. Obviously the best results are obtained with the synergy between a healthy and balanced diet such as the Sirtfood diet and an active lifestyle and healthy sporting activity. However, the effects of Sirtfood diet are already amazing taken alone.

By combining a diet rich in Sirt Foods with an initial moderate caloric restriction, this diet will allow you to lose an average of three pounds in seven days while preserving and even developing your muscle mass.

You see, it is not easy to find good diets for weight loss, yet it is not hard at all. All you have to do is get the right information on what Sirtfood diet is, how it works and its benefits, and the desire to change your current obese lifestyle too much better one.

For that reason, consider staying healthy with Sirtfood diet plan. Sirtfood diet is a well-balanced diet that you will have the benefit of preparing, and it comes with many health lessons. Do not be left out; stay healthy with the Sirtfood diet!

Are you ready to do it for yourself?

In this book, you will discover the science-based details of the Sirtfood diet plan, how it works in our body and our cells (and what it has to do with our DNA!) and its unique properties, as well as benefits, menus, recipes, and questions and answers.

Evolution and nutrition:
parallel or distant roads?

In the last years a growing debate on food and nutrition and about what the good rules of nutrition are or should be has been developed. A key point that should always be taken into consideration when we discuss about these topics is our DNA.

Maybe I am going to be a little bit technical now, but keep hard and remain with me. At the end, you will really understand why you need to know how our DNA works inside our cells and what this has to do with the food we eat every day. These informations will be our milestones for understanding the science behind Sirtfood diet and how this works. Above all, you will discover how to exploit this knowledge to your advantage in order to modulate the activity of your DNA in your favor, acquiring a leaner physical shape and feeling more energy.

As you know, DNA (deoxyribonucleic acid) is a molecule present in the nucleus of (almost) all our cells. Neurons, fat cells, liver cells, red blood cells, skeletal muscle cells and so on, they all share the same DNA, which is unique and unrepeatable and makes every man, every woman and every single living being, from the smallest bacterium to the biggest blue whale, different from each other. Every individual is one and unique and this is due to his/her/its genome, i.e. all the informations contained in the DNA. Consider genome as a library made of DNA, with many shelves. Without going too much into technical language, in genetics, shelves are those called "chromosomes", and each shelf contains many books. Generally, these books are like instruction manuals, as they contains the real informations employed by the cell to perform its activities. Therefore, every book give some instructions to the cell. Well, in genetics the book are called "genes". We can consider genes as a single information package or instruction manual needed to do something. Human genome contains about 20.000 different genes. Noteworthy, despite every cell of our body contain the same identical genome, different cells activate o inactivate different genes. In other words, they read and employ different instructions manual needed for their work. For example, cardiac cells activate only those genes needed to its activity, which is continuously pumping the blood in and out the heart. Instead, adipocytes (the cells of adipose tissue) activate only those genes needed for synthesis and accumulation of fat in our belly, that we need to survive in times of famine (or to get depressed when the pants bought the last summer do not fit well!).

A pretty mess right? Yet, within each of our cells everything is finely regulated and NOTHING is left to chance! This fascinating world is also not a glass bell that does not communicate outside! Far from it! Indeed there is a continuous interplay between our genes and the environment.

An emerging branch of genetics, called epigenetics, is increasingly showing that our genome is not something fixed, but a very dynamic element that interacts with the environments. The Greek prefix "epi" ("ἐπι" "over, outside of, around") in epigenetics implies features that are "on top of" or "in addition to" the traditional genetic basis for inheritance. In biology, epigenetics is indeed the study of the interaction between the DNA of our genome and the environment.

However, what is this "environment"? Well, environment is the pollution or the fresh air you breathe, environment is the stress due to your boss asking the job done within this evening, environment is the love of your family, environment is the physical activity you do, environment are all the different stimuli your body receives during all of your life, from conception to death. And guess what, environment is also the food you eat! It estimated that an adult eat on average about 1 Kg of food per day. If we take the calculator, considering a life expectancy of 80 years we obtain tens of tons of food passing through our gastro-intestinal tract during our life. Not bad!

You can ask what our DNA has to do with what we are eating at lunch: the truth is that the activity of our DNA is strongly conditioned by what we eat. DNA is dynamic, DNA is not passive to what we eat, and DNA interacts with food. The food is a stimulus that can activate or inactivate genes (instructions manuals) of our genome (library). And this is the key point of Sirtfood diet! Sirtfood diet lays its foundation in the science of epigenetics, and in the knowledge of how some foods or, more precisely, some nutrients present in foods can activate, inactivate or modulate the activity of genes.

Unfortunately, the modern diet has somehow forgotten how to employ food to improve our health. Sadly, many of us eat only to fill themselves and not to feed themselves. This eventually led to the modern disease we all know, such as diabetes, obesity and cardiovascular diseases.

However, in this book you will find a message of hope. Much of the power is in our hands! DNA is not static, we can "hack" it to improve our health and our quality of life, if we know how. So, thank you epigenetics!

The science behind Sirtfood diet is abundant and convincing. In the next chapters, we will discover how some foods named Sirt Foods are a concentrate of nutrients with high healthy and slimming epigenetic potential and which these nutrients are. In addition, we will see how the latter work, particularly how they interact with SIRT1. SIRT1 is a specific protein found in many cells of our body, from the skeletal muscle to the liver and the brain, and its job is to make the mediator between food and DNA. In other words it "senses" specific food-derived molecules (or nutrients) and, in response to them, activates or inactivates genes.

Therefore, SIRT1 is a crucial sensor of our metabolism and our health. The aim of this book is to make you understand how SIRT1 works and how to activate it, making you both discover the mechanisms that activate it and giving practical advice to take advantage of the benefits of Sirtfood diet.

Caloric Restriction:
the secret of longevity

Immortality has been an aspiration of humanity since ancient times, with stories and myths of divinities and immortal beings present in all cultures. Actually, *Homo sapiens* has always tried his best to extend his own life as long as possible, and modern medicine has made great strides in the last decades. If we consider the world wide average, in 1950 the life expectation was below 50 years, today we have largely exceeded 70 years of average life! The last decades has been a revolution! However much of these results have been obtained with intrusive medical interventions and pharmacological approaches. As we all know, drugs are artificial molecules, and all drugs have, unfortunately, side effects. Furthermore, the vast majority of drugs treat diseases but do not prevent them, and as we know well, prevention is better than cure. Therefore, it is important to limit the employment of dugs only in cases of strict necessity and to find other ways to extend our health and the quality of our life.

As you have noticed, I am still not talking about weight loss, lost pounds, body composition and diet to reduce the waist, but I am focusing your attention first on something more basic (and precious): the health.

However, the two arguments (weight loss and health) are actually two sides of the same coin and they should always be considered together. There is no health without an adequate physical shape and there is not an adequate physical shape without health: do not think to an obese simply as a "fat" man or woman! He (or she) is a person who is suffering from a true disease and whose health is compromised. Likewise, an anorexic person is not simply an "excessively thin" man or woman, but a person with unhealthy body composition and metabolism. What I mean is that a person's physical appearance and health should go hand in hand. Unfortunately, this is not always the case: in fact, it may be that a person who has lost weight has achieved this goal in an unhealthy way. How many diets cause weight loss aggressively or unhealthily and induce nutritional deficiencies and food imbalances to the person who follows it! The inevitable consequence is that, as soon as you stops following the diet, the lost pounds are taken up with the interests (the famous "yo-yo effect"), throwing us into despair and making us to think that it is useless to try, no diet works.

Nevertheless, in ancient times, the fatty belly was not a big issue for people. People were not so fat, however they lived much less than the third millennium people. Thus, methods to bring longevity benefits have been of much interest throughout history and many societies, including the Ancient Greeks and Romans, have recognized the efficacy of food limitation to extend longevity.

This kind of diet, more precisely called "caloric restriction" (or "dietary restriction"), is a dietary regimen that provides a limited amount of food which is reduced of at least 70% of the calories of an ad libitum diet.

Nowadays, after a number of scientific studies carried for more than a century, we can assert that caloric restriction is one of the most reproducible way to extend the lifespan of mammals. Even if the first studies have been performed in animals different from us, such as yeast, worms and flies, successive studies in mammals (mice and rats) have been very convincing: the researchers found out that feeding rats with a diet containing 20% indigestible cellulose, dramatically extended mean and maximum lifespan of the animals. From this and other studies in mammals, and more recently also in humans, the emerging idea is that caloric restriction is not simply a passive effect but an active one, highly conserved stress response that evolved early in life's history to increase an organism's chance of surviving adversity (*Sinclair, Mech Ageing Dev, 2005*). What does it means? It means that if a body undergoes to a caloric restriction, this body (more precisely, its DNA) senses this as a danger to its own survival and does not act passively just reducing the metabolic and caloric expenditures passively, but it prompts a number of active responses aimed at increasing the chances of survival. For example, under caloric restriction there is an increase of physical activity of the organism. This sounds crazy: you get less food and, in response to that, you increase your body's energy expenditure! However, from an evolutionary point of view, this makes perfect sense: in the primordial world of our cave ancestors, increasing the physical activity in response to caloric restriction meant increasing the chances of obtaining food by looking for and harvesting berries and tubers or hunting game with greater impetus. Moreover, a number of scientists have proposed that caloric restriction imposes a low-intensity biological stress on the organism, and that this elicits a defense response that helps protect it against the causes of aging. The term "hormesis" refers to beneficial actions resulting from the response of an organism to a low-intensity stressor such as caloric restriction. In other words, low caloric intake is a mildly stressful condition that provokes a survival response within the organism, helping it to survive adversity by altering metabolism and increasing the organism's defenses against the causes of aging (*Sinclair, Mech Ageing Dev, 2005*).

As I have already mentioned, NOTHING is left to chance in our DNA and everything makes sense somehow. In this case, caloric restriction represents the environment that modifies how the DNA works and that induces intra-cellular changes responding to the low-intensity biological stress.

There would be enough material and scientific studies to write an entire book about the epigenetic effects of caloric restriction. However, in our case we just need to know that caloric restriction induces the expression of the so-called longevity (or survival) genes within our cells, leading to:

1. Increased antioxidant capacity. Antioxidants are molecules that protects us from damage exerted by free radicals. Free radicals are naturally produced within the body (even this is not totally correct, we can considered them as the garbage of our metabolism) and they can cause damage to our membranes, our proteins and even to our DNA. Antioxidants act as a shield against free radicals.

2. It stimulates the consumption of fats as a source of energy (fat oxidation).

3. It has positive effects on insulin sensitivity. Insulin is a hormone secreted from pancreas that helps to regulate the blood glucose level (glycemia) in animals by lowering glycemia when there is a condition of hyperglycemia.

It seems all very tempting and, indeed, it is! Who would not want to find a way to increase the own health and at the same time lose weight, increasing fat consumption and improving insulin sensitivity? Well, accordingly to scientific research it seems that caloric restriction should be a very effective method.

The Dark Side of Caloric Restriction

If caloric restriction seems to have an outstanding efficacy to support our health and fitness, we can ask ourselves: why so few follow this kind of dietary regimen? Why so few doctors and dieticians suggest to their patients this approach?

The answer is not so easy, probably because there are many reasons. If we want to summarize very quickly the reason why calorie restriction is not so popular nowadays is because of the fact that this approach is not for everyone, it cannot be followed continuously and it must be done very carefully.

First of all, we must consider the psychological aspect of a dietary regimen. A person cannot stay forever under caloric restriction. If from the biological point of view it is possible (even if not for all), from the mental point of view caloric restriction is really difficult, for third millennium people even more. Nowadays, indeed, the possibilities to find something to eat are many, among all the delicacies that we have at home in the fridge and in the cupboard, but we have also the possibility of having *take-away* food for dinner without the effort of cooking, bars, restaurants, street food. Wherever we go, we have the possibility to eat something. Food has not only a nutritional role but also a "pleasure" role. Cooking can become a stimulating and sometimes funny activity, and having lunch or dinner with your family or friends is an occasion for socializing and for being happier. Here, taking food away becomes a serious obstacle to the psychological benefits of food in people attempting fasting or under prolonged caloric restriction with the result that they eventually surrender and give in.

The sustainability reason (what a sad life fasting or dieting forever!) is not the only problem of caloric restriction. Indeed, there are many reasons why caloric restriction, especially if continuous, goes from "advantageous" to "disadvantageous".

Primarily, caloric restriction can lead to one or more deficiencies of one or more essential nutrients for our diet and our health (for example vitamins, minerals, proteins). People undergoing to caloric restriction must be very careful not to miss any of these nutrients, and the task is not so easy without a technician who can help them (e.g. a doctor, a biologist nutritionist or a dietician). If something goes wrong this will involve a decrease in health conditions, with consequent less daily energy, chronic fatigue, a greater difficulty (if not impossibility) in reaching one's own weight and, not least, health problems!

Noteworthy, the risk of nutrients deficiency is even more likely today than few centuries ago! In fact, if we compare the beginning of the last century with today, a hundred years ago foods were more natural and more genuine because they have not undergone industrial processes aimed at increasing its shelf life and often passed directly from the producer to the consumer. They also contained on average more vitamins, minerals and other nutrients than today. Nowadays, with advent of the industrial revolution, large retailers and cold chain always mediate the arrival of food to our kitchens, and many different kinds of industrial treatment are carried out on food matrices. Furthermore, the transport of foods across the oceans and thousands of miles has become normal. Who knows how much time has passed since the harvest, how far has been and what kind of treatments has undergone the tomato I found yesterday at the supermarket!

As a thumb of rule, we can assert that when foods undergo industrial treatments, they lose part of their nutrients.

Furthermore, too intense or too long caloric restriction can compromise our skeletal muscle. The skeletal muscle is not only the organ that allows us to stand, walk, run and hold in hands this book, but it is a fundamentally for our health and for the achievement (and maintenance) of our healthy weight. The skeletal muscle is, in terms of volume, the most abundant organ in our body and is extremely rich in mitochondria, the energy centers of our cells in our body. It is fundamental to have a healthy muscle to have enough mitochondria that can generate energy from carbohydrates and fats as an energy source. In other words (and simplifying a little): more muscle means more active mitochondria inside the skeletal muscle cells, and more mitochondria means more energy expenditure and consumption of fats and carbohydrates, making the aim of being fit and having a slim physique easier.

In order to have a good muscle mass, make sure to include a training program in your week. It is not important which sport you do, the important thing is that you do something that you like doing and that you can do with constancy. This will you keep going to the gym or out for jogging or whatever making you active and your muscles moving and in health. Moreover, make sure to include proteins in your diet.

As you will see in the next chapters, Sirtfood diet suggest including some specific foods (the Sirt Foods) in your diet. Apart from a few exceptions (such as soy or buckwheat), Sirt Foods are not particularly abundant in proteins. Therefore, it is a good choice to combine the properties of Sirt Foods with a good weekly protein intake.

Take note that not all proteins are the same. A steamed mackerel is not the same as a grilled sausage! In the former the good proteins are together with other healthy nutrients such as minerals and essential polyunsaturated omega-3 fatty acids (which are good for your health), while the latter is stuffed of saturated fatty acids (which accumulates in the arteries) and contains toxic substances produced by the grill cooking method.

Good healthy proteins sources are, for examples: lean meat (e.g. chicken, turkey and other poultry), eggs, fish, Greek yogurt, ricotta, legumes (such as soya, beans, peas, chickpeas, lentils). In the case of legumes take into account that the latter contain also an important amount of carbohydrates, so remember it if you are wishing to be low in carbohydrates in your diet.

In conclusion, it seems that caloric restriction, even if in theory could be a good choice to lose weight a live healthier and longer, in practice it encounters a number of obstacles that make it difficult for everyone to tackle.

So what can we do? Do we give up and continue to eat as we always have done losing this opportunity?

Luckily, an alternative allows us both to lose weight staying healthy and to eat with pleasure enjoying the pleasure of food. However, to get there, we must first meet and get to know the magical world of sirtuins, the "skinny genes".

Hints from the yeast

The first steps in the identification of the molecular mechanisms and the gears that govern the complex biological response to caloric restriction, comes from observations on budding yeast *Saccharomyces cerevisiae*. About 20 years ago, researchers found that a specific protein, named Sir2, is determinant of lifespan in yeast cells. Indeed, the expression and activity of Sir2 slowed down ageing and extended lifespan of yeast cells, while yeast cells lacking of this protein died earlier (*Kaeberlein et al., Gene Dev, 1999*). Noteworthy, the extending lifespan effects of dietary restriction in the yeast was abrogated in absence of Sir2, meaning that the latter mediates effects of dietary restriction (*Imai, Cell Biochem Biophys, 2009*).

The molecular key that opens the benefits of calorie restriction was discovered!

From these pioneering observations, several others were made, always with the same results: from flies to worms (the model organisms used in biomedical research), the analogs of Sir2 always extended the lifespan, in the same way caloric restriction does.

Sirtuins and SIRT1

At the beginning of the third millennium scientists were looking forward to taking the next step and to study in human cells whether what happened in yeast and other model organisms was applied to humans too. The excitement over the possible implications was evident!

Now we know that Sir2 belongs to the family of "sirtuins". From the biochemical point of view, sirtuins are "NAD+ dependent protein deacetylases". However, for us is more than enough to acknowledge them as a class of proteins highly conserved in all the organisms, from bacteria to humans, and that these proteins are crucial regulator of ageing, metabolism and, as we will discover in this book, healthy weight loss too.

Sirtuins are very ancient molecules in animal evolution, meaning that their functions are crucial for life and survival. Furthermore, they possess a highly conserved structure throughout all kingdoms of life: in other words, sirtuin of *Saccharomyces cerevisiae* yeast (Sir2) is very similar to sirtuins of other species, from worms to mice until humans. Most likely this means that sirtuins among different species have the same (or very close) function(s). Thus, if Sir2 extends lifespan and slows down ageing in yeast, it is very likely that human sirtuins do the same!

Whereas bacteria and microorganism encode either one or two sirtuins, mammals (*Homo sapiens* included) possesses seven sirtuins (SIRT1, SIRT2, SIRT3, SIRT4, SIRT5, SIRT6, and SIRT7). However, the most important and the most interesting mammal sirtuin is SIRT1.

SIRT1 (whose name stands for "silent mating type information regulation 2 homolog 1") is the mammal sirtuin whose function is the most similar to Sir2 of yeast, and thus the one most studied in the recent years.

SIRT1 is present in many compartment of our body, ranging from skeletal muscle to adipose tissue, as well as in other organs, such as liver, heart and brain. In the cells of these tissues, it occupies two different compartments: the cytoplasm, which is the peripheral part of the cell, and the nucleus, which is the cell "command room" where DNA is present and operates. More precisely, SIRT1 shuttles between the cytoplasm and the nucleus: in the cytoplasm, it waits for informations from the environment and, when it receive them, it moves to nucleus. We will see later which kind of environmental stimuli activate SIRT1 to move from cytoplasm to the nucleus and to do its job. In the nucleus,

SIRT1 acts as an epigenetic regulator: it is indeed able to change how DNA works and express by means of activating or inactivating specific genes of the cell. The result is a change of cell activity and functions.

SIRT1 plays a crucial role in the metabolism and physiology of our body: it acts as a key epigenetic mediator that coordinates metabolic responses to nutritional availability in various tissues. As its homolog Sir2 does in yeast, SIRT1 has a lifespan-extending effect.

Let's see where and how SIRT1 acts. Remember, the basis of Sirtfood diet are the functions of SIRT1 and how to activate them.

I will try to be not too technical but, trust me, understanding the true science behind Sirtfood diet is really important to be master of our own nutrition and lifestyle, and not a simple followers of this or that diet.

SIRT1 in skeletal muscle

As already mentioned, SIRT1 is a protein found in many districts of the organism and its activities result in increasing lifespan and slowing down ageing. Many of these activities can be exploit to achieve healthy weight loss, i.e. reduction of fat mass without affecting muscle mass. As we have seen earlier, muscle mass is extremely important both for general health and for maintaining a slim shape.

In the skeletal muscle, SIRT1 is particularly active and ready to receive inputs that prompt its activity. Once activated in myocytes, SIRT1 exert two main tasks.

First of all, SIRT1 switch the kind of fuel employed by the muscle: it decreases the oxidation of carbohydrates and increases the use of fats for energy purposes. Usually, carbohydrates, under the form of glucose or glycogen (the reservoir of glucose in the muscle), are the fuel of first choice and fats are used ("unfortunately" for us) with greater difficulty. This is the reason why the fatty belly is so difficult to eliminate. This is too an evolutionary mechanism of survival: for our cave ancestors it was very important to accumulate fats into the adipose tissue (or fat tissue) and not to employ it as a source of energy during times when food was available. The fat accumulated was a source of energy of crucial importance for survival during lean times. The problem is that today lean times do not exist anymore (at least in the western world) and the fatty belly has become a health problem and no longer a survival mechanism. Therefore, the activity of SIRT1 is very useful in this context to induce the bigger organ of our body to consume the exceeding fats.

The second activity of SIRT1 in the skeletal muscle is strictly linked to the first one. In order to be "burned" and employed as an energy substrates, fatty acids must enter a sort of cellular furnaces, that use them and "burns" them in the presence of oxygen (hence the name of fat oxidation). These furnaces are mitochondria. Imagine mitochondria like many "little beans", covered by two membranes, spread through the cytoplasm, burning glucose or fatty acids as a source of energy and producing ATP, the organic compound which provides the energy needed for the many processes of living cells. The activity of SIRT1 is to increase the number those little beans, thus raising the fat oxidation capacity of the skeletal muscle. SIRT1, indeed, stimulates the activity of another protein, PGC-1 alpha, which is the master regulator of production of new mitochondria.

Finally, it has been reported that, in myocytes, SIRT1 contributes to the improvement of insulin sensitivity. Insulin is a pancreas-derived hormone that regulates blood glucose levels (i.e. the glycemia) (*Imai, Cell Biochem Biophys, 2009*). In few words, insulin "says" to our cells to take up glucose from the blood when the glycemia is too high (i.e. hyperglycemia). This finely regulated mechanism is necessary to maintain glycemia within a specific concentration range, not too low, not too high. Chronic hyperglycemia (blood glucose continuously too high) is noxious to health and is the first step towards diabetes mellitus. SIRT1 helps insulin to work properly, making the entry of glucose into cells more effective and preventing situations of uncontrolled hyperglycemia.

DID YOU KNOW that proteins are macronutrients of crucial importance in promoting health? All the fundamental biomolecules of our organism are made of or by proteins (such as antibodies, enzymes, neurotransmitters, contractile proteins and so on). The best proteins for our health are those from animal sources, as they contain a higher amount of essential amino acids. Essential amino acids are those amino acids our body is not able to produce, and therefore must obtain from the diet. Some essential amino acids are able to support SIRT1 activity in heart and skeletal muscle (*D'Antona et al., Cell Metab, 2010*).

To summarize, once activated in the muscle SIRT1 increases the number and the activity of mitochondria, the energetic furnaces of our cells that "burn" fat and it helps to better control glycemia.

SIRT1 in adipose tissue

Before analyzing what SIRT1 does in the adipose tissue, we must first point out two important notions.

The first one is that adipose tissue is not simply a "warehouse" of fatty acids (and a source of extreme sadness if there is too much of them!) but it is an active organ interacting with other organs and tissues. In particular, it secretes a number of hormone that regulates the physiology of our organism. One of the most important is adiponectin. Adiponectin is a very good ally to lose weight as it combats obesity and diabetes, enhances insulin sensitivity, and promotes proper glucose homeostasis. Adiponectin is produced and secreted by the adipose tissue during caloric restriction and exercise. Accordingly, lean people produce more adiponectin in their adipose tissue than overweight people do. Recent studies has also shown that adiponectin induce SIRT1 activation, thus indicating a molecular mechanism linking caloric restriction to SIRT1 actions.

Secondly, we must take into account that there are different kinds of adipose tissue: white adipose tissue (WAT) and brown adipose tissue (BAT) are the main ones. BAT is abundant in small mammals and in newborns and helps them to survive to cold temperatures, while WAT is more prominent in adults. The main function of the WAT is to store excess energy in the form of fat, whereas BAT is specialized to dissipate energy as heat. BAT it is therefore of particular interest ad it dissipates energy by burning fatty acids.

Now we have explored some of adipose tissue secrets, let's see what SIRT1 does to it.

Firstly, SIRT1 induce fat mobilization in WAT by repressing PPAR-gamma (Peroxisome proliferator-activated receptor gamma). PPAR-gamma (don't be scared by the name!) is one of the master gene that drives fat storage in white adipose tissue (*Picard et al., Nature, 2004*). By repressing it, SIRT1 reverses the trend and stimulates the release of free fatty acid form WAT to the blood. From here, free fatty acids will be driven to the different organs (especially the skeletal muscle: do you remember the increased fat oxidation in myocytes under the influence of SIRT1?) where they can be employed as a source of energy.

Further, SIRT1 can induce WAT to switch into metabolically active BAT! It is very amazing that SIRT1 is able to transform the metabolic inert WAT into the energy-burning BAT, thus increasing the caloric expenditure thorough the day. Noteworthy, it seems that reducing WAT levels increase lifespan, as it was observed that mice with reduced levels of it live longer (*Picard et al., Nature, 2004*).

SIRT1 in the liver

Liver is one of central command center of our metabolism. After receiving stimuli from different districts of our body, it builds new molecules useful for the body's functions and destroys those no longer necessary or potentially harmful.

In the liver, SIRT1 regulates cholesterol metabolism and decreases synthesis of LDL, the so-called "bad" cholesterol (it is named "bad" because it tends to accumulates in the walls of arteries inducing atherosclerosis and other cardiovascular diseases). It also activates the reverse cholesterol transport, a process that in which the liver cleanses excess cholesterol throughout the body by reabsorbing it.

Meanwhile, to increase energy production, SIRT1 stimulates fatty acid oxidation in the liver too and, at the same time, blocks synthesis of new fat molecules.

SIRT1 in the brain

One of the most unexpected effects of caloric restriction observed by researchers was the increase of physical activity level when food availability was low. As already mentioned, this makes sense from the evolutionary point of view as it prompts the organism to move to action in search of sources of food. In 2010 it was made light on the mechanism by which increased physical activity and energy expenditure was induced by caloric restriction. Guess who is the player? Still SIRT1, this time acting in the brain, more precisely in the hypothalamus. The latter is an area deep inside the brain, it is important for coordinating many basic activities including feeding, body temperature, energy expenditure. SIRT1 levels in the hypothalamus change in response to diet, and during caloric restriction SIRT1 level increases, promoting higher physical activity and increasing body temperature with a resulting increased body energetic expenditure (*Satoh et al., J Neurosci, 2010*). Moreover, SIRT1 activity in the hypothalamus is protective against obesity and diabetes, as mice devoid of SIRT1 in the hypothalamus neurons are more susceptible to these diseases.

SIRT1 in the heart

One of the most frequent age-associated disease is atherosclerosis, which is caused partly by chronic inflammation in the blood vessel. With aging, the lack of regeneration and defense from free radicals strongly compromise the function of blood vessels. SIRT1 activity in blood vessels is able to reduce the accumulation of atherosclerotic plaques. Moreover, SIRT1 activity has ability to lower blood pressure. SIRT1 has been demonstrated to be vital in maintaining cardiac health too, as it increases myocardial ischemic tolerance and protects against hypertrophy. In the heart, it also stimulates fat oxidation (*Chang & Guarente, Trends Endocrinol Metab, 2014*).

How to activate SIRT1

We have just seen the many activities of SIRT1 in many of the districts and organs of our body. I make you note that what I said to you is only a small part of SIRT1 job. I decided to focus only on those tasks that can be useful for healthy weight loss and to fight aging and aging-related diseases. Furthermore, remember that humans, like all mammals, have seven sirtuins and SIRT1, even if the most important, is only one of them. Other sirtuins have important functions in our organism too, and many of them work in synergy with SIRT1. In addition, scientific research in this field is really pushing hard trying to discover new pieces of the puzzle and it is likely that in the years to come new informations about SIRT1 and other sirtuins will be revealed.

What I want to make you understand is that the situation is elaborate and much more complex of what we have seen. However the take home message remains. SIRT1 is a very important regulator of our metabolism and can be very helpful in keeping us fit.

The beautiful thing is that SIRT1 and other sirtuins are epigenetic mediators. As mentioned before, this means that SIRT1 is a sensor of what happens in the environment and in the specific case of sirtuins they senses the food availability. SIRT1 is like a little soldier ready to receive orders from his captain. The soldier stands ready for the order and when he receive it, he rapidly goes to the command center to communicate the information. Like the soldier, SIRT1 receive informations relatively to food shortage. In a body subjected to caloric restriction, the soldier-SIRT1 take this information and goes to the nucleus (the command center) to say to DNA to change its gene expression and to respond adequately to the situation of caloric restriction. This involves all the metabolic changes and all SIRT1 actions previously analyzed. We have seen that SIRT1 inhibits fat storage in the adipose tissue and induce the latter to send fatty acids to other organs for burning them and that SIRT1 speeds up fat oxidation in the skeletal muscle, in the liver and in the adipose tissue too, inducing the proliferation of the energy-consuming brown adipose tissue (BAT). SIRT1 increase the basal metabolic rate (the energy spent during the day) by increasing the number of mitochondria in the muscle and acting directly in the brain. Moreover, SIRT1 actions exert protection against some aging-related diseases such as diabetes, obesity and cardio-vascular diseases and lower cholesterol too. Indeed, a number of reports have also demonstrated that mice with high levels of SIRT1 can mitigate disease syndromes much like caloric restriction, including diabetes, neurodegenerative diseases, liver steatosis, bone loss and inflammation (*Chang & Guarente, Trends Endocrinol Metab, 2014*).

Wonderful! The next question then is the following: how do we activate SIRT1?

We have already mentioned part of the answer: caloric restriction is an effective way to induce SIRT1 activation. The reduction of calories available to the organism is a signal that SIRT1 interprets and transfer to DNA and genes. However caloric restriction is not a good idea for everyone nor for long times and it should be undertaken under medical advice or, in any case, with the help of a professional in the sector. In addition, caloric restriction requires great sacrifices and restrictions and is therefore very difficult to follow, especially from a psychological point of view.

Another way to activate SIRT1 is physical activity. It is know that during the effort SIRT1 can be activated (we will see better in the next chapters the molecular mechanisms by which SIRT1 is activated during physical activity) and it is know that people with low fat mass has a better capacity of SIRT1 activation than overweight people. This is due, at least partly to the higher production of the hormone adiponectin, which activates SIRT1, in the body of lean and physically active people. Conversely, a high fat diet can trigger the loss of SIRT1 action in mice, and obesity can reduce the expression of SIRT1 in humans (*Chang & Guarente, Trends Endocrinol Metab, 2014*)

If, after these considerations, you are wondering if there are no alternatives to going on a diet and doing physical activity every day, wait and follow my reasoning.

A fundamental question we must ask ourselves is the following: are all the beneficial effects of caloric restriction mediated by SIRT1 or also by other effectors that we do not know? If this were the case, we would have to resign ourselves to eating less. But if, instead, the main effector of caloric restriction were SIRT1 and we found an alternative way to activate SIRT1, then we would have found another way to take advantage of the wonderful beneficial actions of SIRT1 without fasting! This would be wonderful! Let's see what science tells us. First of all, it has been reported that mice without SIRT1 are metabolically inefficient and unable to adapt to caloric restriction normally. Secondly, mice without SIRT1 do not show the usual increase in physical activity induced by caloric restriction. Most revealingly, mice lacking SIRT1 do not live longer on a caloric restriction diet!

From these pivotal observations, we can truly say that SIRT1 is the crucial sensor, mediator and effector of caloric restriction. Amazing! Now we just have to find a way to activate SIRT1 that is different from caloric restriction. The pharmaceutical industry is trying to find a molecule that recognizes and pharmacologically activates SIRT1. However the results so far are very poor and, in any case, we know that the use of drugs must always be limited for their side effects and because they are artificial substances recognized as not own by the body and that must be disposed of in some way, usually in the liver. We would need something provided by nature itself, to which our body and our DNA has been accustomed over the centuries and millennia of human history and capable of activating SIRT1.

A natural substance with this effect seems impossible to find, yet it has always been with us. Indeed, I will say more, there is not only one substance like this but there are many!

Do you think I am drunk? Well yes and no...

The secret of SIRT1-activation without fasting comes from studies... on red wine!

Red wine: the first Sirt Food
and the clinical studies on resveratrol

Vitis vinifera

Let food be thy medicine,

And let medicine be thy food

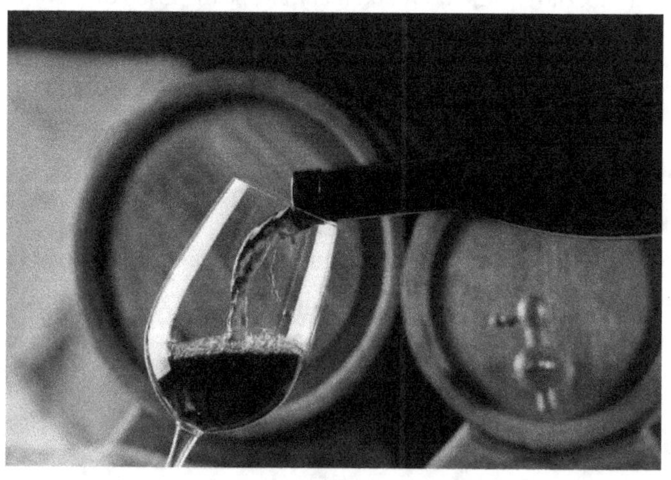

This is one of the most famous quote of Hippocrates of Kos, the Greek physician that lived between the fourth and third century BC, and one of the fathers Sif medicine. Actually, this quote is one of the most famous quote of medicine itself, as well as of science of nutrition.

In other words, Hippocrates meant that food contains some molecules (the nutrients) that can induce positive changes in our body, inducing a greater state of health and well-being. Without knowing anything about genetics, Hippocrates had laid the foundations of the epigenetic role of food in our health: depending on what foods (or what nutrients) we provide to our body, the latter (through our DNA) will evoke biological actions in response to the former.

Do you follow a diet rich in sugars and saturated fats? The epigenetic response will results in a constant and intense increase in blood sugar, followed by a hyper-reaction of the pancreas that will secrete more and more insulin, leading, over time, to insulin insensitivity and eventually diabetes. Meanwhile, excess saturated fat will accumulate in the arteries and blood vessels leading to atherosclerosis. This is epigenetics.

Do you follow a healthy and balanced diet, containing all the nutrients necessary for the functioning of our body? The glycemia will be under control and your blood vessel will be free from atherosclerotic plaques. Your health will benefit and your body will thank you. This is epigenetics.

Much of our health is, as you can see, in our hands, when we buy food in the supermarket, when we cook or when we order a dish in the restaurant.

The quote of Hippocrates had to be well present in the mind of a group of researchers from the Harvard Medical School, Boston, while they were looking for natural molecules with the ability to selectively activate sirtuins and SIRT1 in a pharmacological-like way, but without the side-effects of artificial drugs.

The amazement of the scientists was certainly great when the results of their analyzes indicated that not only they had identified one food-derived sirtuins-activating molecule, but 6 different ones! All of them were able to activate Sir2, the analog of SIRT1, in the cells of the yeast *Saccharomyces cerevisiae* and, by doing this, to increase cell survival and yeast lifespan! These discoveries revolutionized the knowledge of anti-aging processes and the scope of the research was such that it was published in *Nature*, the most important and prestigious international scientific journal, in 2003 (*Howitz et al., Nature, 2003*)!

In the study, the most potent activator of SIRT1 was resveratrol, a nutrient found in red wine and black grapes, which is associated with a surprising number of health benefits, most notably the mitigation of age-related diseases, including neurodegeneration and atherosclerosis.

From a chemical point of view, resveratrol is a polyphenol.

A polyphenol is a natural molecule of vegetable origin (animals do not produce them). As the name implies (poly-, meaning "many", and phenol), a polyphenol is a relatively complex molecule made up of multiple units of phenol. I do not want to go into too much detail about the magical world of chemistry; anyway, a phenol is essentially a small, "round-shaped" molecule containing carbon, hydrogen and oxygen. Resveratrol contains two phenols inside it, one at one end of the molecule and one at the other end (as shown in the following figure).

*Polyphenols group: Polyphenols constitute a family of about 5000 organic molecules widely present in the plant kingdom. They are characterized, as the name indicates, by the presence of multiple phenolic groups associated in more or less complex structures. **Top Left:** Phenol, the single unit of which all polyphenols are constituted; **Top right:** Resveratrol, a polyphenol abundant in red wine; **Bottom Left:** Quercetin, a polyphenol present in many vegetal food, such as capers, apple, celery; **Bottom Right:** Epigallocatechin Gallate (EGCG), one of the most abundant polyphenol in tea, especially in green tea.*

More than 5000 different molecules belong to the group of polyphenols, and many of them can enter our body through food. It is well known and recognized that polyphenols are good for health, and until 2003 this was attributed only to their antioxidant power (in some polyphenols quite high).

DID YOU KNOW that browning of apples and of many other vegetables is due to oxidation of polyphenols? Polyphenols, when exposed to the air oxygen, react with the latter and oxidize to form the dark-colored molecules that we see, for example, in an apple cut in half and left in the air. These dark molecules are named melanins and are the same responsible for our tan when sunbathing, even if in this case they are not produced from polyphenols. A particular enzyme present in plants, called "polyphenol oxidase", speeds up the oxidation reaction between polyphenols and oxygen present in the air. As the reaction of the polyphenol oxidase is speeded up by heat and oxygen, you can leave the apple cut in half in a closed, cool container in order to reduce the oxidation of polyphenols and the browning of the half-cut apples (or other fruits and vegetables).

However, we now know that many of the positive effects attributed to resveratrol and its "friends" polyphenols are due to their ability to activate SIRT1 and other sirtuins.

For example, other SIRT1-activating polyphenols identified in the 2003 study were: piceatannol (a polyphenol similar to resveratrol than can be found in red wine and black grapes too), isoliquiritigenin (found in liquorice and soy), fisetin (contained in strawberries, apples, onion, cucumbers and other vegetables), quercetin (particularly abundant in capers, but rich also in onions, tea, wine, apples, forest fruits, buckwheat, kale, celery and other vegetables) and butein. Collectively, polyphenols able to activate SIRT1 were named "caloric restriction mimetics".

Nevertheless, among the known SIRT1-activating polyphenols, resveratrol certainly has a prominent position, as one of the most powerful SIRT1-activator.

Resveratrol is particularly abundant in the skin and seeds of black grapes (*Vitis vinifera*) and in red wine (the alcoholic beverage obtained from the fermentation of pressed black grapes) too.

The beneficial effects observed in yeast were also replicated in human. In a 2011 study, obese humans received resveratrol supplementation to their diet for 30 days. In muscle cells, SIRT1 was markedly activated, this induced metabolic changes mimicking the effects of caloric restriction: improved fat oxidation and consumption, decreased hepatic lipid content, better glycemia control, and dropped systolic blood pressure (*Timmers et al., Cell Metab, 2011*).

Therefore, we can truly say that we have found a method to activate SIRT1 without necessarily fasting or running two hours in a row on the treadmill! Black grapes and red wine are therefore our first Sirt Food. A Sirt Food is a food that, thanks to its nutritional properties (the particular polyphenols contained), is able to activate SIRT1 and to induce the beneficial actions of SIRT1 that we have seen previously.

Actually, that red wine was a special food is nothing new and was recognized well before the study by Howitz and colleagues in 2003.

The history of wine goes back to prehistoric times; it is so old that it is confused with the history of humanity itself. The oldest evidence of serial wine production was found in Armenia (about 4,100 BC, more than 6000 years ago!), with the discovery of the oldest existing cellar when drinking culture likely involved ceremonies in honor of the dead.

The temporary altered state of consciousness attributable to the intake of wine (commonly known as drunkenness) was considered in a religious context from its origins. In the Ancient Greece, Dionysus was worshiped and the Ancient Rome transmitted its cult through the figure of Bacchus. Wine is still considered today a symbol of conviviality associated with its consumption in the circle of family and friends.

Its etymology is probably related to the Latin word "*vis*" (strength) because one of its functions was to "increase the strength of body and soul ".

Hippocrates himself prescribed wine to treat wounds, as well as antifebrile, purgative and diuretic drink. The wine continued to have great therapeutic use also in the Roman Empire and in the Middle Ages too. But it was Arnaldo da Villanova's "*Liber de Vinis*" ("Book about wine", 13th century AD) that firmly established the use of wine as a recognized therapeutic tool. Among the extensive list of its medicinal uses, the book underlined its antiseptic qualities. There was also an important aspect, more practical, but equally useful for the doctors of the time: throughout the medieval period, wine was one of the few liquids capable, due to its alcohol content, of dissolving and hiding the flavor of substances, sometimes with disgusting tastes, and it was considered curative by the doctors of the time.

From a chemical point of view, wine is mostly water (more than 80 % of weight). The fermentation produces ethanol (the molecule contributing to the alcoholic grade of wine) as well as other secondary metabolites of fermentation, such as glycerol. Glycerol is particularly viscous and thanks to this property, you can observe it directly in the glass of wine, when you swing the wine itself in the glass and in the upper part there is a viscous halo that slowly descends from the walls of the glass: that is glycerol. Wine also contain acids (such as tartaric acid and malic acid) and a sugar residue (most of it is used during alcoholic fermentation) which contribute to the taste of wine, as well as aromatic compounds. Noteworthy, polyphenols in wine have a better bioavailability than grapes. In fact, maceration of full grapes (with skin and seeds included) and alcoholic fermentation allow extraction of polyphenols into the wines (*Garrido-Banuelos et al., Food Chem, 2019*). The concentration and composition of phenolic compounds impact also the flavour and mouthfeel of wines.

According to science, the therapeutic effects of red wine, if taken in moderate doses (a glass of per day), are due to polyphenols, present mainly in red wine.

However, many of you may think that wine contains alcohol, which is toxic to our cells. In any case, there is a trick that we can use to exploit the good properties of resveratrol and other red wine polyphenols, avoiding the possible damage (especially to the liver) of alcohol. In fact, if we cook our dishes (for example a braised beef dish) with red wine, we are able to eliminate the alcohol, which evaporates completely in the heat, keeping the resveratrol molecules and other polyphenols intact. Perfect trick! Your dishes will benefit in taste and aroma too. Of course, sometimes we can treat ourselves to a glass of red wine, which can really be an explosion of pleasure for our taste buds. Now we can do it with less guilt, as we know now that the resveratrol contained in it is a strong activator of SIRT1. Obviously, moderation in the intake of red wine and alcohol contained in it must be the rule. Nevertheless, we now know that other Sirt Foods exist and we can combine them in a number of ways to compose our Sirt Food Diet plan!

Now can meet all other Sirt Foods other than red wine now, discover their secrets and their wonders.

Let's take a look!

SIRT FOOD	MAIN SIRTUINS-ACTIVATOR CONTAINED
Red Wine and black grapes	Resveratrol, Piceatannol
Bell peppers and Chili Peppers	Luteolin, Myricetin
Buckwheat	Rutin
Capers	Kaempferol, Quercetin, Rutin
Celery	Apigenin, Luteolin, Kaempferol
Cocoa	Epicatechin
Coffee	Caffeic Acid, Chlorogenic Acid
EVO Oil	Oleuropein, Hydroxytyrosol
Matcha Tea	Epigallocatechin gallate (EGCG)
Kale	Kaempferol, Quercetin
Lovage	Quercetin
Medjoul Dates	Gallic Acid, Caffeic Acid
Parsley	Apigenin, Myricetin
Red Chicory	Luteolin
Red Onion	Quercetin
Arugula	Kaempferol, Quercetin
Soy and derivatives	Daidzein, Formononetin
Strawberries	Fisetin, Quercetin, Kaempferol
Apple	Epicatechin, chlorogenic acid, Quercetin,
Turmeric	Curcumin
Walnuts	Gallic Acid

(Adapted from Goggins & Matten, The Sirt Food Diet, Yellow Kite, 2016)

Sirt Foods

Bell peppers and Chili Peppers: different brothers

Capsicum spp.

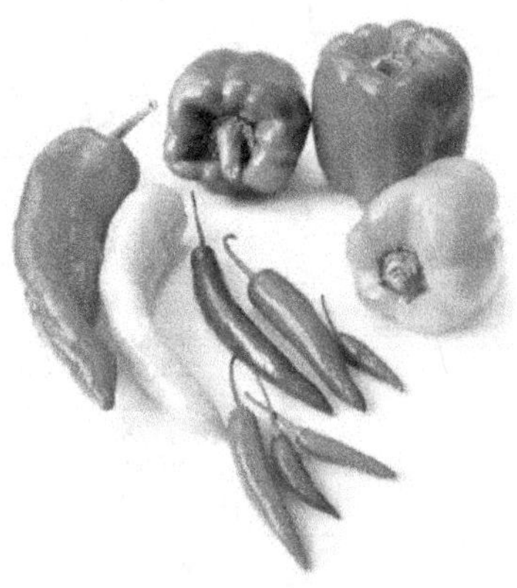

Bell peppers and chili peppers are one of the most amazing gift brought by Christopher Columbus from the New World to Europe. So close from the botanical point of view (they belong to the same genus: *Capsicum*), so different in sizes, colors and shapes. The most important difference between bell peppers (also known as sweet peppers) and chili peppers is the spiciness, absent in the former and present (sometimes infernal!) in the latter. This is due to a genetic mutation that happened to bell peppers, which lost the ability to produce capsaicin, the spicy molecule that is, instead, abundant in chili pepper. The degree of spiciness can be measured empirically through the Scoville scale.

Actually, chili pepper is not only one specie but a group of five different species, which share the same botanic features and the ability to synthetize capsaicin: *Capsicum annuum, Capsicum frutescens, Capsicum chinense, Capsicum baccatum* and *Capsicum pubescens.* Bell pepper is a variety of *Capsicum annuum.* According to some, its scientific Latin name "*Capsicum*" derives from "*capsa*", which means "box", referring to the shape of the fruit (a berry) which resembles a box with seeds inside. Others derive the term from the Greek "*Kapto*" which means to bite, with evident reference to the spicy sensation that bites the tongue while eating. From the testimony of archaeological finds, we know that as early as 5500 BC it was known in the area of the present-day Mexico. The Aztecs used chili peppers in their religious rituals and they already knew many of its therapeutic properties: it made digest better and it was useful against rheumatic pains. Now we know that chili peppers is also a good help in weight control: indeed it reduces appetite and it is thermogenic, which means that its nutrients, especially the spicy capsaicin, activates basal metabolic rate, making the body consume more calories during the day. It is also a good friend of the arteries as it promotes microcirculation through the activation of peripheral flow.

DID YOU KNOW that the color of the pepper is not connected, as many think, to its spiciness? There are completely green varieties that are much spicier than other red varieties. The spiciest chili pepper variety of ever has been established to be the Carolina Reaper (obtained the first time from hybridization between a Red Habanero and a Naga Morich originally from South Carolina) by Guinness World Records in 2013.

Also bell peppers are an important guardian for health: the remarkable presence of vitamin C makes them a product with various healthy characteristics, primarily antioxidants. The presence of beta-carotene is also very relevant, especially in red pepper; it contains various B vitamins and many minerals, mainly potassium, but also iron, magnesium, calcium.

Despite the differences between them, the two brothers share a good content of SIRT1-activatin polyphenols, in particular myricetin and luteolin.

DID YOU KNOW that capsaicin, the spicy substance the chili peppers, is irritating to eyes and mucous membranes? If you have worked in the kitchen struggling with chilies, avoid touching your eyes or any type of mucous membrane or open wound. In addition, when you go to the bathroom, remember to wash your hands, not only after but also before! Water and soap do not completely remove the capsaicin from the fingers, but the former is reduced thanks to the mechanical action of rubbing.

Buckwheat: besides the name there is much more

Fagopyrum esculentum

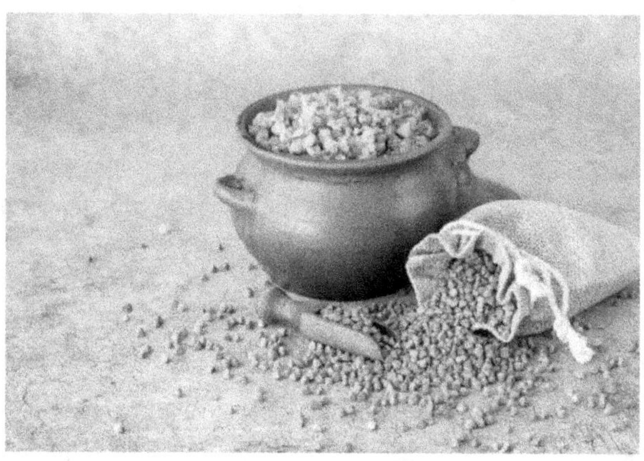

Rustic, resistant to cold climates and difficult to attack by parasites, buckwheat has very ancient origins. Its cultivation begins in the areas of Siberia, Manchuria and China. Over time, buckwheat also begins to be grown in Japan, India and Turkey. It then landed in Italy in the fifteenth century, thanks to maritime trade across the Black Sea, and only after the Middle Ages it acquired a distribution and cultivation worthy of note at European level.

Despite its name, this seed is not a cereal, and it does not belongs to this family. It is often referred as pseudo-cereal (as, for example, quinoa and amaranth). Indeed, as other pseudo-cereals, buckwheat is naturally gluten-free and can therefore be included in the gluten-free diet of people with this condition. It has excellent nutritional qualities and it is particularly rich in minerals such as iron, zinc and selenium. It is also an excellent source of vegetal proteins (>12 g per 100 g) with an high biological value: unlike most cereals, it has in fact a good content of lysine, an essential amino acid generally lacking in vegetal foods. Moreover, buckwheat is characterized by a low-glycemic index due also to the good amount of fibers, making this food particularly suitable to people with diabetes or low insulin sensitivity. Finally, the polyphenol content is high and the **SIRT**1-activating rutin is particularly abundant: until 20 mg of rutin per 100 g (*Kreft et al., J Exp Bot, 2002*).

Capers: the cargo of quercetin

Capparis spinosa

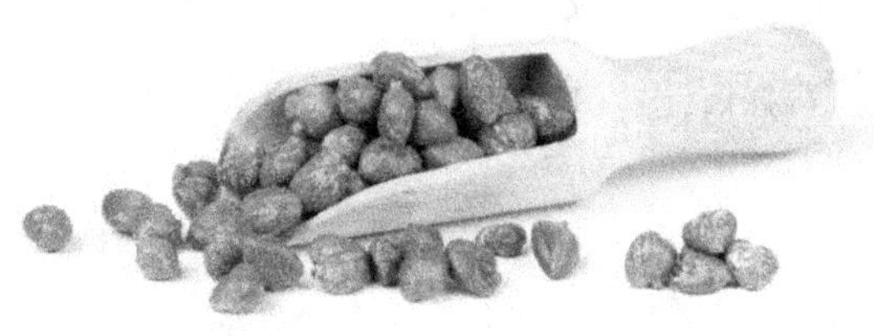

A joy for the taste buds, capers are the buds of the homonymous plant (*Capparis spinosa*) widespread in the Mediterranean area since immemorial time. The wide diffusion in the Italian island Sicily and the traditional use that is made of it in Sicilian cuisine have led capers to be included in the list of traditional Italian agri-food products. The aromatic properties are contained in the flower buds, that are harvested when they begin to bloom between end of May and first of September: indeed in that time flower buds are not yet opened and sprouted. Fresh capers are very bitter and unpleasant. Therefore, every day at the end of the harvest, the capers are placed in a vat, they are covered with abundant coarse sea salt and mixed for about ten days. The water emitted and the salt that dissolves form a brine that makes them mature.

Capers are extremely rich in polyphenols that are able to activate **SIRT1** activity. They are also particularly abundant in rutin, keampferol and (take note) they are the food with the highest quercetin content in relation to the weight! In few words, they are small, delicious, tasty polyphenols cargoes!

Celery: an ancient fresh remedy

Apium graveolens

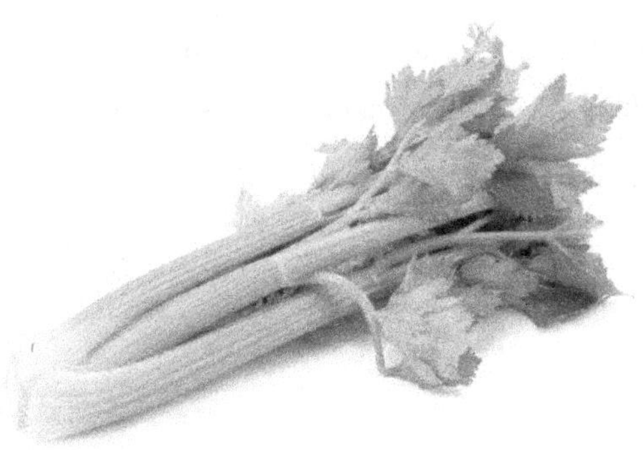

Celery was a sacred plant for the Hellenics. Hellenics abstained from using celery in the kitchen as a common ingredient, because they believed it was a sacrilege towards an exceptional plant. Homer himself attributed divine properties to it, as evidenced in the passage in the Iliad where Achilles heals his horse from serious illness thanks to celery.

For its digestive, stimulating, fortifying and anti-rheumatic virtues, celery juice was among the remedies of the ancient pharmacopoeia. Hippocrates (460–370 BC), the Father of

Medicine, stated: "For the upset nerves, celery is your food and remedy."

In ancient Rome instead celery was used abundantly in the kitchen, and even during banquets they prepared crowns for diners, since they thought that its aroma would counteract the alcoholic intoxication.

As the "interpretations" of celery have been so different in the great cultures of ancient times, as various are the possible uses of celery in today's kitchen. They goes from the fresh celery (it is wonderful in the *pinzimonio* or in all kinds of salads) to the employment as an ingredients in soups and stews, where it emphasizes the sweetness of meat, fish or seafood.

According to various studies, among natural compounds, celery is one of the most important sources of phytochemicals such as antioxidants such as vitamin C, beta-carotene (Provitamin A), manganese and SIRT1-activating polyphenols: apigenin (of which celery is one of the richest foods), luteolin, and kaempferol.

Among the properties attributed to celery the anti-inflammatory action and protection against cardiovascular diseases, in particular atherosclerosis, stand out.

Dark Chocolate: the food of the Gods

Theobroma cacao

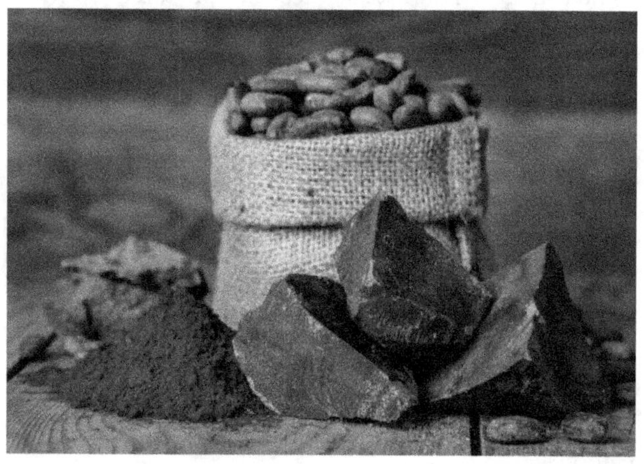

The story of chocolate is one of the most fascinating stories regarding origin of a food. As we all know, chocolate is produced from dried and fully fermented fatty seeds of cocoa plant (*Theobroma cacao*). This plant takes its name from a word of proto amerinda origin pronounced "*kakawa*". The first farmers who started cultivating the plant were the Maya around 1000 BC, making chocolate one of the oldest food in history, now consumed all over the world.

The name of the genus, *Theobroma*, indicated by Charles Linnaeus in the 18th century, derives from ancient Greek and means "*Food of the Gods*". Indeed already ancient people of Central America knew the numerous healing properties attributed to cocoa. The seeds were a symbol of prosperity in religious rites; a medicine capable of healing the diseases of the mind and body (erythema, diarrhea or stomach pain) was based on cocoa. Noteworthy, cocoa seeds were the basis of the monetary system! A cocoa seed was worth the equivalent of four corn cobs, three seeds were used to buy a pumpkin or a turkey egg, and with one hundred you could get hold of a canoe or a cotton cloak!

From a chemical point of view, cocoa powder is the food with the highest content of polyphenols (up to 50 mg of polyphenols per gram), and it is an excellent source of antioxidants and minerals (especially magnesium, copper, potassium, and calcium). The polyphenols are responsible for the bitterness of cocoa powder. The main polyphenol found in cocoa are epicatechin and catechin. In addition to polyphenols, cocoa contains methylxanthine compounds, predominantly theobromine.

In virtue of all these precious nutrients man health benefits have been associated to cocoa consumption: anti-inflammatory activity, reduction of risk of diabetes by optimizing insulin sensitivity. Moreover some studies suggest cocoa polyphenols protect nerves from injury and they protect also the skin from oxidative damage from UV radiation (*Katz et al., Antioxid Redox Sign, 2011*). Approximately 70 human intervention studies have been carried out on cocoa and cocoa-containing products. These studies indicate that the most robust biomarkers positively affected are endothelial function, blood pressure, and cholesterol level, making of cocoa powder a healthy choice for your heart (*Ellam & Williamson, Annu Rev Nutr, 2013*). Of course, dark chocolate containing >85% cocoa is strongly preferable, in virtue to higher content of cocoa powder and thus polyphenols and other healthy nutrients. Avoid milk chocolate!

Coffee: the king of healthy beverages

Coffea spp.

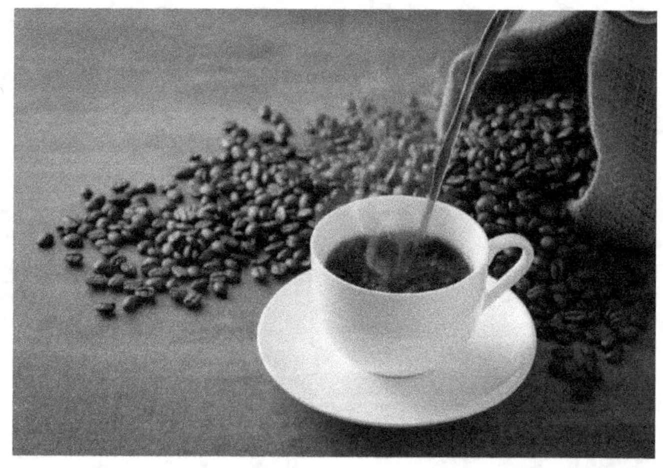

Probably one of the most famous, consumed and appreciated beverage all around the world, coffee is a drink obtained by grinding the seeds of some species of small tropical trees belonging to the genus *Coffea*.

The discovery of the use of fresh fruits from the coffee tree probably dates back to around the 9th century AD in Ethiopia, where nomads chewed them raw or prepared an energetic and stimulating decoction.

The coffee tree is a small evergreen shrub. The ripe fruits are of a garnet red color, similar to cherries, and contain two green beans, sticked together. There are two main botanical varieties: "*Arabica*" that comes from Central America, more valuable and aromatic; "*Robusta*", of Central African and Asian origin, more bitter but less expensive. The Coffee powder is made after roasting the beans.

The conquest march of the coffee from Ethiopia toward all the World, however, was not without obstacles and contradictions. Muslim origins pushed the clergy to formally ask to Pope Clement VIII for the prohibition of coffee consumption. The legend says that the Pope would have blessed it and then he had pronounced the following: "it is so exquisite that it would be a shame to let it be drunk exclusively by the infidels".

The coffee has a very complex aroma given by the great variety of substances (over 800 compounds), most of which are formed during the bean roasting process. One of them is chlorogenic acid. Recent research revealed that some of the mechanisms of healthy effects of this polyphenol is due to activation of SIRT1, which in turn promotes proper mitochondria function and prevents LDL-cholesterol to aggregate and to induce atherosclerosis (*Tsai et al., Mol Nutr Food Res, 2018*). Chlorogenic acid exert also an antioxidant effect and may have a role in slowing down glucose release in the blood after a meal. Of course, remember that this effect is nullified if you pour half a pound of sugar into the coffee cup!

Coffee is also a natural anti-depressant (don't you feel more enthusiastic after a good coffee?) and the caffeine (a natural molecule belonging to the family of alkaloids and particularly abundant in coffee) contained can speed the burning of fat by acting directly on adipose tissue.

DID YOU KNOW that caffeine and theine are... **synonyms??** Caffeine is present in many different plants and, during history, it took the name from the botanic source. Caffeine and theine are therefore the same molecule (1,3,7-Trimethylxanthine) with different names! Similarly, caffeine can also be called guaranine if it comes from guarana (*Paullinia cupana*), a typical plant of the Amazon rainforest.

Noteworthy, a meta-analysis published in 2017 has finally demonstrated that coffee is truly good for your health! The study indicates the coffee consumption (3-4 cups a day) is associated to reduction of risk of cardiovascular mortality and cardiovascular disease, and is associated with an 18% lower risk of incident cancer (*Poole et al., BMJ, 2017*). Similar results were obtained also with decaffeinated coffee, indicating that the effect is not mediated by caffeine but by other molecules contained in the beverage.

Nevertheless, if you suffer from hypertension, remember not to overdo coffee and that you can take it decaffeinated.

DID YOU KNOW that caffeine is a great help for your workout? According to the position stand of the International Society of Sport Nutrition (ISSN) caffeine consumed in low/moderate dosages is effective in improving the sport performance, by increasing vigilance sustaining maximal endurance exercise and stimulating the basal metabolic rate (*Goldstein et al., JISSN, 2010*).

Extra Virgin Olive Oil:
the secret of Mediterranean diet

Olea europaea

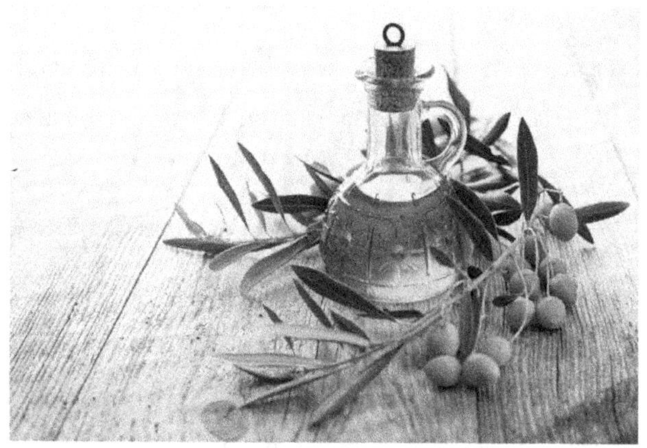

Olive oil is a food oil extracted from olives, or the fruits of the olive, a tree of Mediterranean origin. In Greece olives were used to produce oil from at least 4000 years ago. Nowadays the most important producers of olive oils are Spain, Italy and Greece, however olives are also grown outside the Mediterranean, thanks to the properties of its oil, which is highly appreciated for its flavor. The olives intended for the production of the oil are the ripe ones, which begin to change color from green to purple/black: at this time, in fact, the content of aromas and oil is maximum.

DID YOU KNOW that the fruity aromas characteristic of a good oil extracted from olives are produced only when the olives are mechanically crushed? If you smell a whole olive you do not feel the same aromas of a good extra virgin olive oil. The aromas of oil are in fact the result of enzymatic processes that begin with the pressing phase of oil production. Specific enzymes, previously enclosed in special vacuoles inside the cells, are released following the mechanical breakage of the latter during the pressing phase. These enzymes in turn produce new volatile molecules that can disperse in the air and reach our nose receptors, giving rise to those magnificent characteristic aromas of olive oil.

Olive oil is distinguished from all other edible oils by its peculiar flavor and by the high content of oleic acid, a monounsaturated fatty acid with beneficial effects on the cardiovascular system. Olive oil has few saturated fatty acids and a high content of unsaturated fatty acids (in particular monounsaturated and a small portion of polyunsaturated)

The virgin type is obtained from the mechanical pressing of olives, without the use of solvents. In olive oil can also be present (in low quantity) free fatty acids. The latter have a bad smell, can interacts and damage other molecules present in the oil and they reduce oil thermal stability, so it is very important to keep their content very low in the final product. Virgin olive oils are those with free fatty acid content lower than 2%, while Extra virgin olive (EVO) oils are those whose free fatty acid content is below 0,8%.

Therefore, purchasing EVO oil guarantees an oil that has kept the original properties of the olives to the higher level, including the polyphenols they contain.

Among the latter, oleuropein is the main polyphenol present in olive oil and it is the main nutrient responsible for the bitter taste of olives and its oil. It has antimicrobial, fungicidal and insecticidal activity, acting as a plant defense against infections and infestations.

Oleuropein has beneficial properties for numerous diseases such as neoplasms, cardiovascular diseases, diabetes and neurodegenerative diseases. These properties are not limited to the known antioxidant power of polyphenols; more recent studies have, in fact, started to demonstrate the effective clinical efficacy on humans given by the interaction between oleuropein and SIRT1 and its functions. We can be sure that the future will reveal other pleasant surprises about olive oil, the secret of one of the healthiest diet ever, the Mediterranean diet.

Matcha Tea: an infusions of polyphenols

Camellia sinensis

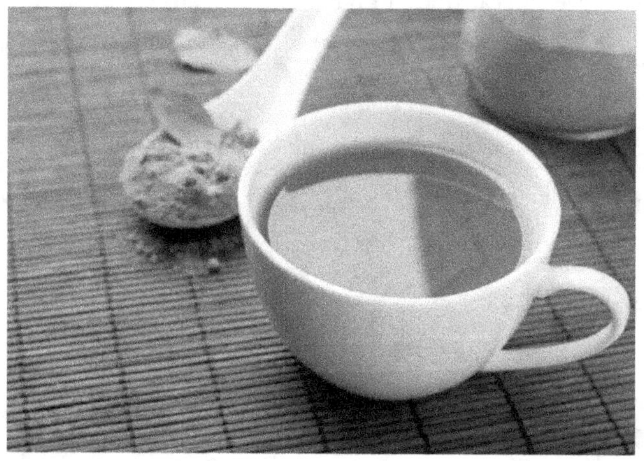

Matcha tea is the famous Japanese tea of excellent quality and bright green color, produced from the leaves of *Tencha*, a particular type of green tea that is processed and chopped to obtain Matcha powder.

Despite the popular belief, this tea originated in China, where it was consumed during the famous tea ceremony since the 8th century AD. The preparation and consumption of this delicious tea then became part of the Buddhist Chan ritual. According to tradition, it was a Buddhist monk of the Tendai sect, Saicho, who introduced the drink to Japan at the beginning of the 9th century AD. Three or four centuries later the Zen monks did not fail to drink a large bowl of Matcha (powdered green tea rich in vitamins) before facing long hours of meditation.

Production of Matcha tea requires Tencha leaves to be covered with dark nets before the harvest in order to strongly reduce the sunlight that reaches the plant. This pushes the plant to produce large amounts of chlorophyll (which gives the bright green color to matcha tea), a higher percentage of antioxidants (the highest among the different types of tea, even higher than normal green tea) and theanine. Theanine is a very particular nutrient acting directly on brain, being neuroprotective and inducing relaxation; theanine combines with the caffeine contained in tea reducing its side effects and producing a state of alert relaxation: so it gives you the same energy without the sudden crash due to excessive caffeine consumption. That's why it is said that caffeine in matcha and green teas is different from caffeine in coffee. Actually, this is not true: the caffeine is the same, but in green tea the effect is modulated by theanine.

After about 20 days of shadow, Tencha leaves are ready to be harvested by hand-picking. The artisanal process of making tea from leaves takes a long time and this process makes it so unique. The Matcha stone grinding process lasts no less than an hour for 40 grams of product!

For all these reasons, Matcha tea is counted among superfoods and functional foods. Noteworthy, it contains also polyphenols, epigallocatechin gallate (EGCG) the most important and abundant, which has powerful antioxidant properties, even 20 times stronger than Vitamin E, and quercetin too.

In Addition, Matcha tea is great for maintain your healthy weight. A recent study observed that matcha green tea drinking enhances exercise-induced fat oxidation in humans (*Willems et al., Int J Sport Nutr Exe, 2018*).

DID YOU KNOW that green tea is a good ally for the control of glycemia? Drinking green tea may help decrease blood sugar levels. In fact, one meta-analysis found that drinking at least 3 cups (237 mL) per day was associated with a 16% lower risk of developing diabetes (*Yang et al., BMJ Open, 2014*).

Kale: the king of green leafy vegetables

Brassica oleracea var. sabellica

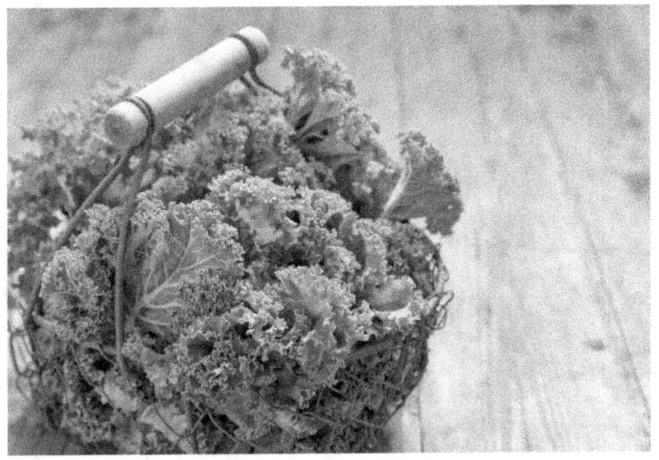

Kale is a specific variety of cabbage (*Brassica oleracea*) one of the most nutritious foods we have.

Curly kale is an excellent source of Vitamin C. Vitamin C (ascorbic acid) is a water soluble antioxidant that is needed for many functions in cells (for example, it is needed to synthesize collagen, the most abundant structural protein in the body). Kale contains more Vitamin C than many other vegetables, much more than an orange.

Kale is rich in beta-carotene (which is transformed into vitamin A) into the body and lutein and zeaxanthin. These nutrients are very important (even if not only) for the health and function of eyes.

> **DID YOU KNOW** why kale and cabbage have a bad smell? This is because they are vegetables rich in sulfur compounds which are released during cooking. Try cooking them in the pressure cooker, in order to reduce both the cooking time a lower diffusion of bad smells.

Moreover, kale is one of the best sources of Vitamin K1, a micronutrient essential for blood clotting (a process needed, for example, to close wounds).

Like other vegetables belonging to *Brassicacee* family (i.e. arugula), kale contains a high content of the SIRT1-activating polyphenols quercetin and kaempferol.

Adding kale to own diet is relatively simple: you can add it to the salad, stir-fry it or to prepare centrifuges and smoothies.

Lovage: the secret of monks

Levisticum officinale

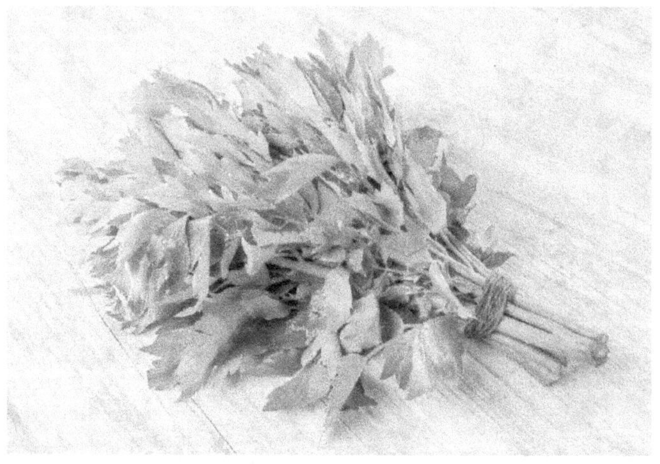

Even if little known, nevertheless, lovage (or "mountain celery") absolutely deserves its place among the magnificent Sirt Foods. For some reasons this perennial plant is rarely used in western cuisine, even if in the history has occupied an important role both in cooking and in traditional medicine, from the Ancient Rome to the Middle Age. Thanks to Benedictine monks, who cultivate it in their 'simple garden' together with other officinal plants, the knowledge about lovage properties (such as calming pain, antispasmodic and diuretic) has been explored and expanded.

Lovage leaves are similar to those of celery (hence its second name "mountain celery"). Its flavor is similar to celery too, but with a much more intense and more pungent aroma which makes it very pleasant. Lovage is ideal both raw in mixed salad and as condiments for risotto and soups.

Thanks to its properties, it is also widely used in the preparation of herbal teas, especially for diuretic purposes.

Regarding polyphenols content, lovage is very rich in the SIRT1-activating quercetin, whose content is second only to capers!

Medjool dates: the superfood from the East

Phoenix dactylifera

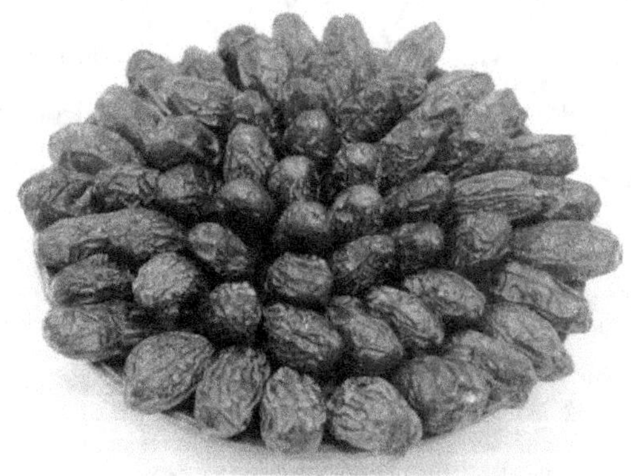

The date palm is the classic symbol of an oasis, and has played an important role for ancient human settlements (for at least 7000 years) in the deserts of the Middle East, North Africa and north western India. Considered the first plant cultivated by humanity, it begins to bear fruit only after the eighth year of life, reaching full maturity at thirty years. Already in ancient Egypt it was a tree appreciated for its very energetic fruits. Dates can be eaten both fresh and dried.

Dried dates are darker than fresh ones and with wrinkled skin and are more caloric than fresh ones.

The 'Medjool' date is a specific cultivation with bigger fruits than other dates and particularly sweet and tasty. Originally from Morocco, it is now cultivated also in Israel and other states of Middle-East once belonging to Fertile Crescent. Medjool date were introduced into the American continent at the beginning of the 20th century in Southern California in the United States. At the end of the 1960s, the 'Medjool' was brought to northern Mexico, in the San Luis Rio Colorado Valley in the State of Sonora and later into the Mexicali Valley in the State of Baja California, becoming the main date cultivation grown in Mexico. These two valleys accounted for 97% of date production in Mexico for the year 2017.

The Medjool cultivation has distinct advantages over other cultivations, such as high yields, high quality fruits and high nutritional value: analysis of the minerals revealed that the most abundant element for the pulp is potassium (even more than bananas), 0.85 g per 100 g (*Salomón-Torres et al., PeerJ, 2019*). The high potassium content reduces the risk of stroke, heart attack and other heart pathologies. Consuming regularly dates can help to lower the level of LDL cholesterol and, thanks to the presence of magnesium, which regulate high blood pressure. The potassium contained in Medjool dates is also very useful for to the functioning of the nervous system.

There are numerous reports about the high concentration of phenolic acids in the date, and specifically a higher concentration in the seed, giving it a great antioxidant potential (*Salomón-Torres et al., PeerJ, 2019*).

Remember: due to the high content of carbohydrates (>60%) dates are energy-dense food, so do not exceed with them. They are optimal before going jogging or before a workout or, also, as a mid-morning/mid-afternoon snack. They are good for sporty people also for reintegrating properties of mineral salts.

Parsley: the omnipresent herb

Petroselinum crispum

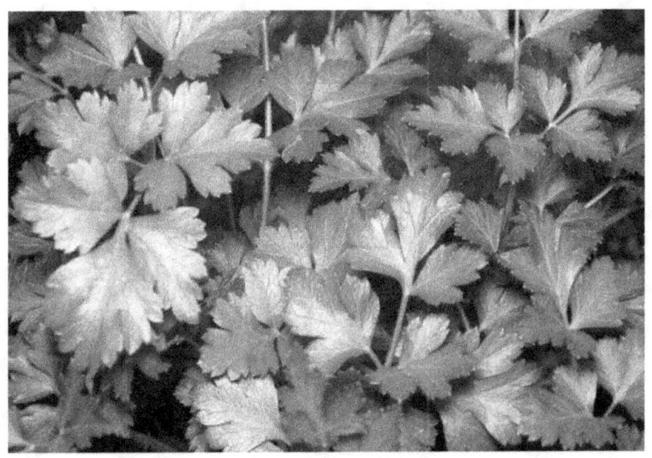

The origin of parsley is from Mediterranean region, but today is cultivated wherever of the world. Parsley can grow both in pots and in the garden and, although suffering from extreme climate (excessive hot or excessive cold), it grows quickly. If the leaves are wilted, once watered it is possible to see them "rise" in a few minutes.

The fresh, green, woody notes of parsley can be combined with many foods in a vast number of recipes ranging from risotto, mushrooms, different types of cooking of meat and fishes. Its herbaceous flavor is ideal for combining it with other herbs too, for example in the salads.

It was in the Middle Ages that parsley gained great popular recognition and utilization. His presence became habitual in the kitchen, hence the motto "being like parsley" to indicate something or someone omnipresent. With centuries, parsley gained also great credit as a medicinal herb.

Parsley is a traditional medicinal plant whose alleged properties have been confirmed by modern medicine, with various proven pharmacological properties including antioxidant, hepatoprotective, neuroprotective, anti-diabetic, analgesic, spasmolytic, immunosuppressant, anti-coagulant, anti-ulcer, diuretic, hypotensive, anti-bacterial and (ok now I'm finished) antifungal activities. Parsley is among the richest food in the polyphenol apigenin (which activates SIRT1), but contains also luteolin, quercetin and kaempferol (*Farzaei et al., J Tradit Chin Med 2013*).

Red Chicory: the sheperds' clock

Cichorium intybus

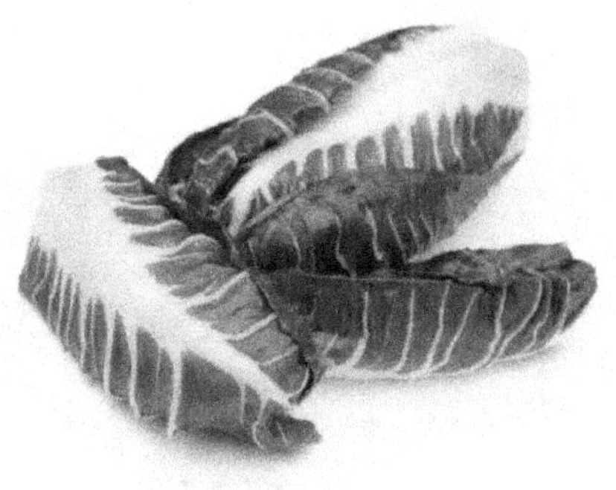

Still in the mid-1900s, chicory was used in gastronomy in soups, in cosmetics in purifying masks, and in herbal medicine in digestive herbal teas. Its flowers have the characteristic of always opening in the morning at the same time and closing in the second part of the afternoon around four o'clock. For this reason, in some areas of the Alps, chicory is called the "shepherds' clock", because usually when its flowers close, the mountaineers milk the cows in the pasture. The red cultivars of chicory are good friends in the sirtfood diet as they contain a number of pholyphenols, such as luteolin and quercetin, known to activate SIRT1 and to reduce chronic inflammation and decrease atherosclerosis. Chicory is also an excellent source of inulin, a prebiotic fiber.

Red Onion: the ancient medicine

Allium cepa

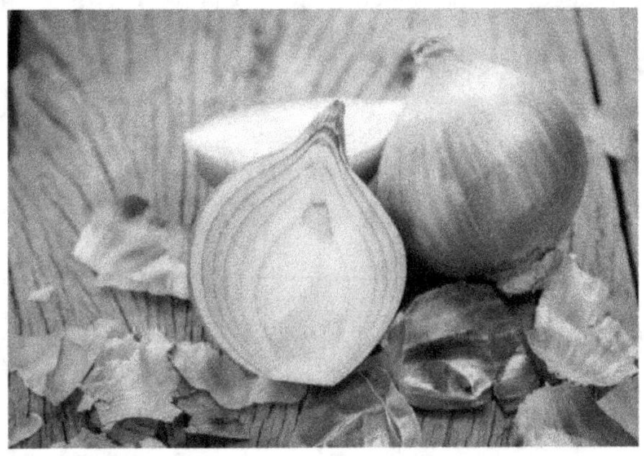

Onion is one of the oldest vegetables among those consumed by human. Native of the Asian continent (Iran or Afghanistan), the onion was known and consumed by the Egyptians since 3000 BC. Onion was represented in the frescoes of the tombs of the pharaohs. It was revered as a divinity and it was called to testify to oaths or put in the hands, on the chest and on the hollow of the eyes of the dead passing to the afterlife.

There are many varieties of onions that can differ greatly in shapes and colors. The edible part of the plant is the bulb In particular, two widespread sub-categories can be distinguished: the white onion and the red onion. The red onion distinguished from other varieties by its sweetness and, indeed, it is employed to making jams. The differences between white and red onion goes far beyond: indeed the red colour of red onion indicates a vast array of antioxidant nutrients, especially the polyphenol quercetin.

DID YOU KNOW that there are remedies for "onion cutting" tears? Over the centuries chefs and housewives have tried all ways to avoid (or at least limit) the tearing effect in cutting the onion. Since volatile molecules trigger the tears and are released when the onion cells are broken by the knife, the goal is to prevent these molecules from reaching our eyes. As the tear factor is well soluble in water, wetting with water the knife and the cutting board is a good way to "trap" the tear factor between the water molecules and prevent it from being released into the air and reaching our poor cornea.

Accordingly, Greek botanist and physician Discorides (40-90 AD) indicated that the white variety was more suitable as a food, while the red one as a medicine. The Roman Physician Galen (129-210 AD) also espoused the same thesis, considering the red color an indication of a more intense curative efficacy.

Arugula (I'm a "rocket" Veg!)

Eruca sativa

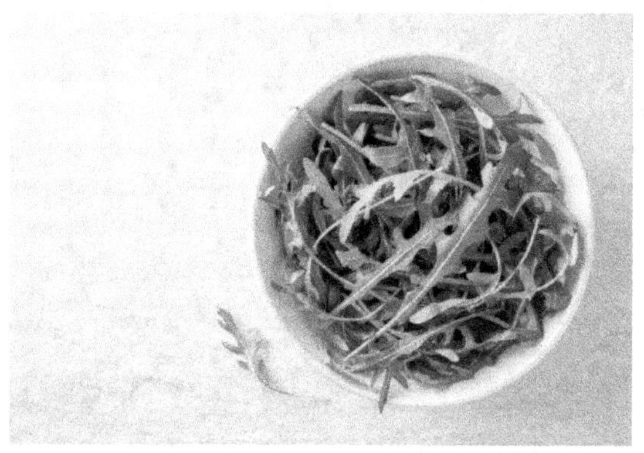

When at the restaurant you find that nice "little herb" put in the plate as decoration element and you don't eat it leaving it in the plate... you should know that not eating it is a mortal sin!

Obviously I am joking, but it is really a pity to deprive yourself of a food so rich in properties (and polyphenols)!

I'm speaking of Arugula, also known as garden rocket, it is one of the most nutritious green-leafy vegetable of

Mediterranean origin. It is a small, low growing annual herb featuring elongated, lobular leaves with green-veins.

The taste of arugula is particularly appreciated as it is strongly aromatic and pungent (slightly spicy). The typical use of arugula is as a side dish, even if it can also be used to make a pesto (pasta sauce). Moreover, a salad with arugula as a main ingredient is perfect for who loves strong tastes.

It seems that the name "arugula" derives from the Latin term "eruca" which means "to burn", perhaps inspired by the pungent and spicy taste of this herb. Moreover, this herb was considered a natural aphrodisiac and it was used in the form of a decoction to combat impotence since ancient times. Actually the research then showed that there is something true, as was shown that arugula is an effective food in the inhibition of an enzyme that causes erection problems in humans, with consequent stimulation of blood supply to the *corpora cavernosa* of the penis (*Alhowiriny et al., J Med Plant Res, 2013*)

DID YOU KNOW that, in the Middle Ages, arugula was ... censored? This fact was due to the sex-stimulating activities attributed to arugula. In the poem "Moretum", probably written by Virgil, we find the verse "et Veneris revocans eruca morantuem" which, translated, means "and the rocket awakens the senses of those who are sleepy". The reputation as an herb capable of stimulating desire accompanied the rocket throughout the Middle Ages, a period during which, precisely for this reason, it enjoyed less luck and its cultivation in convents and monasteries was prohibited because it was considered "herb of lust".

However, as research tells us, arugula has many more health benefits. First of all, arugula is among the richest vegetables in fiber, calcium, iron, potassium, phosphorus, vitamins of all groups, in particular C and group B. precisely because its wide spectrum content of vitamins and minerals, arugula is associated with beneficial and aesthetic properties towards hair, nails and skin. In fact, in situations of deficiency of some micronutrients, the first ones showing signs of it are hair, nails and skin.

Arugula is also a good diuretic and it has antithrombotic actions. It is also particularly rich of the **SIRT**1-activating polyphenols quercetin and kaempferol (*Heimler et al., J Agric Food Chem, 2007*). Last but not least, it has antihypertensive effects for the presence of erucine (a sulfur containing molecule named like this as it is abundant in arugula (*Eruca sativa*).

Soy: the king of legumes

Glycine max

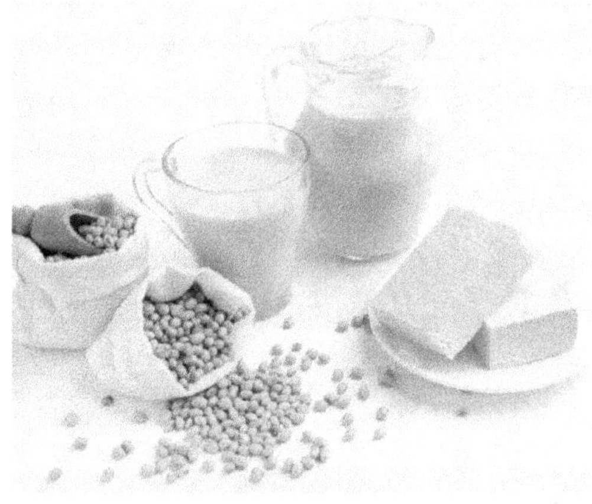

Soy is the legume with the highest protein content (36 g of protein per 100 g of raw weight). It is also a type of vegetable protein with a high biological value, as it contain a high content of essential amino acids (comparable with animal proteins). The lipid content is higher than other legumes, however the quality of these is very good (high content of monounsaturated and polyunsaturated fatty acids). Soy is very rich of minerals too, especially Iron, Magnesium, Potassium, Selenium, Zinc, Manganese.

A great advantage of soy is its cholesterol lowering action, mainly due to the synergistic action of soy lecithin and soy isoflavones. Isoflavones are a particular subfamily of polyphenols typical of legumes and among the most well-known and abundant isoflavones in soy are genistein and daidzein. These substances increase the excretion of cholesterol and, in particular of the so-called "bad" LDL cholesterol, while leaving the "good" HDL cholesterol unchanged, that is, the one with protective action against cardiovascular diseases. It is no coincidence that in the areas of the world where the consumption of soy and derivatives is higher, the incidence of cardiovascular diseases is lower. The relationship causes effect and therefore the beneficial action of isoflavones in heart health was supported by a number of scientific publications as summarized in a recent meta-analysis concluding that the overall evidence indicates that soybean consumption is inversely proportional to the incidence of cardiovascular disease and heart attack. (*Yan et al., Eur J Prev Cardiol, 2017*).

A more recent observational study carried out by the American Heart Association further showed that those who eat tofu and foods rich in isoflavones have a lower risk of going to heart disease (*Ma et al., Circulation, 2020*).

In the study, researchers from Harvard Medical School and Brigham and Women's Hospital analyzed data from over 200,000 people. All subjects, at the time of the start of the studies, had no diagnosis of heart disease and their diet was recorded. The analysis revealed that consuming tofu more than once a week was associated with an 18% lower risk of heart disease, compared with a 12% lower risk for those who ate tofu less than once a month.

DID YOU KNOW that one of the most famous soy preparations of Chinese origin, tofu, can be easily made at home? Tofu is in fact the result of soy milk curd, and can also be prepared at home. Here follows the procedure.

Hydrate soybeans with water and then blend the soybeans together with water (1 liter each 100 grams soybeans) with a blender.

Transfer to a pot and heat the mixture, stirring until almost boiling. Continue stirring for another 15-20 minutes.

Stop the heating and, as soon as the liquid is cold enough to be able to handle it with your hands, pass it into a porous dish cloth or a fine-mesh sieve.

Squeeze well with hands and let out the liquid part, which is the soy milk, separating it from the solid part (named "Okara") left inside the cloth (or on the sieve).

(continues in the next page)

(*continues from the previous page*)

The obtained soy milk can be drunk within a few days (it can be kept in the fridge), otherwise it can be used in the preparation of tofu, in which it is necessary to curdle the soy milk

In order to curdle soy milk, transfer it into a pot and heat while stirring. After a while, before reaching the boil, add the coagulating agent: I recommend the traditional Japanese Nigari (you can easily find it in oriental food stores). Dissolve the contents of about 1 teaspoon of Nigari in about 100 mL of warm water and add about a third of the solution containing Nigari to the hot soy milk, mix, cover the pot for 5 minutes, add again more Nigari, mix, cover the pot again for 5 minutes, until all the Nigari solution is added. Eventually the soy curd will precipitate separating from the liquid part.

Finally, add the curd in a perforated cheese mold and covered it with a dish cloth (alternatively you can separate the liquid from the whey with a fine-mesh sieve), squeeze to make all the liquid come out well. Let it rest.

After about half an hour the homemade tofu is ready to be eaten or stored in the fridge for a maximum of 4-5 days.

Strawberries:
sweety, tasty, healthy non-fruits

Fragaria spp.

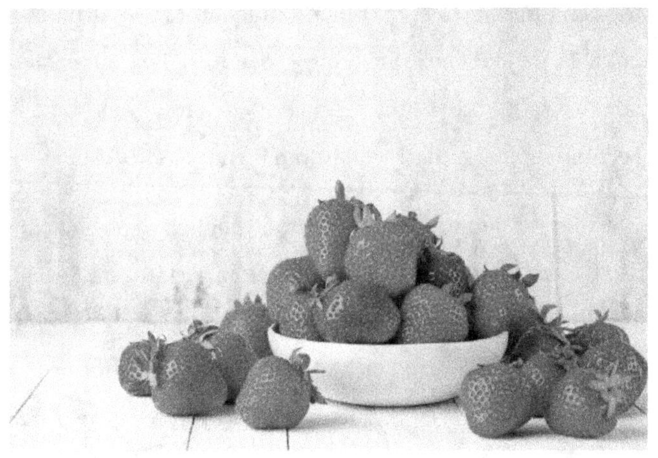

It is certainly the most popular berry fruit in the world, and one of the sweetest ever. When ripe, fresh strawberries reveal a combination of fruity, caramelized and sweet hints with green notes, which make them one of the tastiest fruit nature can offer... even if, truly, it is not a real fruit! Indeed botanically speaking the strawberry is not a fruit: the real fruits are identified in the so-called "achenes", which are the yellow seeds of the surface, and the part of the red and tasty "fake fruit" is nothing else than the enlarged receptacle of an inflorescence.

In ancient Rome strawberries were considered an aphrodisiac and this notion has survived until today through the centuries. Indeed, in contemporary times these fruits are suitable for the amalgamation of love for color, shape and softness. In order to stimulate exciting visions it is recommended to marry them with cream or chocolate.

Strawberries are widely used in confectionery, but since the 1980s, with the spread in Italy of Nouvelle Cuisine, which has upset the traditional concepts of aromatic associations, this fruit has had some luck also as a component of risotto and a sweet and sour sauce created to accompany large roasts and meat dishes. Ultimately, there is no recipe in which strawberries cannot be used or at least tested.

Strawberry has many healthy virtues: first of all, it has a very high antioxidant power, much higher than that of other foods and it is extremely rich of vitamin C, about 60 mg per 100 g fresh fruit, more than citrus fruits (*Giampieri et al., Food & Function, 2015*). That's why strawberry is at the top of the USDA's special ranking of foods that keep young. It is also particularly suitable for fighting the bad cholesterol. Strawberry also is used for laxative, diuretic and purifying, refreshing, diuretic, purifying and detoxifying properties. Finally, they contain xylitol, a sweet substance that prevents the formation of dental plaque and kills the germs responsible for bad breath.

> **DID YOU KNOW** that vitamin C is a "fragile" vitamin? Vitamin C (ascorbic acid) is crucial for our health. Unfortunately, vitamin C is quite unstable and can be damaged by heat, light and oxygen. In the intact fruit or vegetable, vitamin C is safely protected into the cells. However, when the food is manipulated (e.g. it is cooked with heat or an orange juice is prepared) vitamin C can be exposed to heat, sunlight and air, thus being partially lost. So, when you order an orange juice at the café, make sure it is freshly prepared!

In addition to traditional nutrients, strawberries are among the richest dietary sources of polyphenols! The major class of strawberry polyphenols are anthocyanins, ellagitannins and the **SIRT1**-activators quercetin, kaempferol and fisetin. Noteworthy, recent studies has demonstrated for these molecules present in strawberries exert neuroprotective effects, reduction of hypertension and other cardio-vascular pathologies risk and even anti-cancer activity (*Giampieri et al., Food & Function, 2015*).

It is also important to underline the fact that many of the nutritional and health-promoting properties of strawberries are also present in its close relatives wild berries (blueberries, raspberries, blackberries and others). So sometimes it is nice, healthy and fun to vary between these fruits and experiment with their countless applications in your recipes.

Apples: one a day keeps the doctor away (...and SIRT1 active!)

Malus domestica

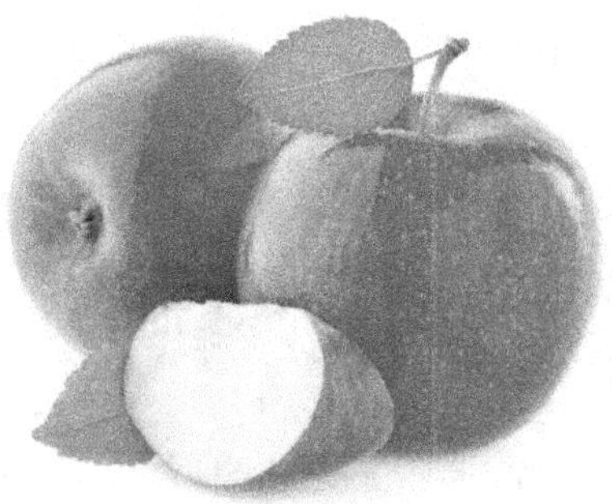

Apple is one of the most iconic food of history: from the apple of Adam and Eve to the apple of Snow White and the apple of William Tell or Isaac Newton and many other stories. It is evident that the apple has played a very important role in the culture of peoples along centuries, not only on a nutritional level but also on a symbolic level. Apple is not only a food but also much more: it is a marvelous symbol of nature differentiation: it is estimated that all the different apple cultivars existing in nature (even those not edible) are about 7000!

Originally from Central Asia where it was grown already in the Neolithic period, the apple spread across the Middle East, first in Egypt along the Nile valley and, subsequently, in Greece. Thanks to the conquests of the Roman Empire, he arrived in the West and from here, throughout continental Europe. The modern varieties of apples derive from only four ancestral varieties that came into contact thanks to the exchanges along the ancient Silk Road.

The apple is one of the food with the highest antioxidant power. This is due to the vast array of micronutrients contained: not only vitamins (provitamin A, vitamins B1, B2, B3, B6, B9, E and C) but also carotenoids and polyphenols. A complete discussion of all the apple polyphenols is very difficult to deal with, mainly because among the different varieties of apples existing there is a great diversification in terms of polyphenols produced in the fruit. However, a study published in 2018 shed more light on the content of the different polyphenols in some representative cultivars, both in the peel and in the pulp (*Kschonsek et al., Antioxidants, 2018*). Among the most abundant SIRT1-activating polyphenols in apples that can be found roughly in all cultivars, we can find quercetin, chlorogenic acid and epicatechin. Apples are also rich in procyanidins, a group of polyphenols. It is still not clear if procyanidins activate SIRT1 or not (some studies say yes but they are preliminary). However procyanidins (in particular procyanidin B2) have be shown to be effective in lowering LDL-cholesterol and promoting hair health by fortifying hair bulb.

> **DID YOU KNOW** that you should not discard the apple peel? In fact, most of the most interesting nutritional compounds are concentrated in the apple peel, including most of the polyphenols. In addition, the peel contributes effectively to satiety thanks for the fiber contained.

Turmeric and curcumin:
the protection from the nature

Curcuma longa

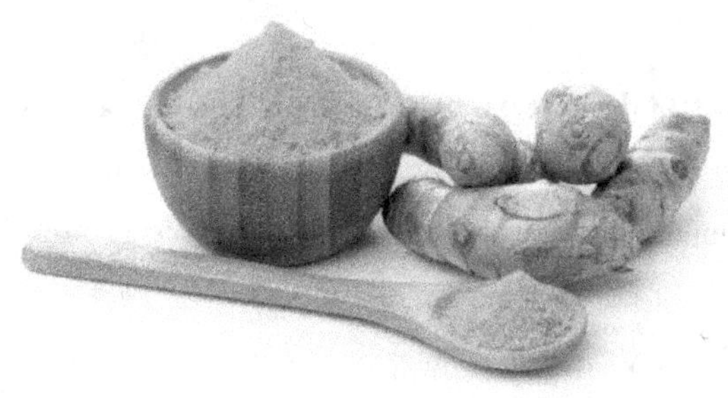

If there is a food known in the field of functional medicine since hundreds of years ago, this is turmeric (*Curcuma longa*), a herb belonging to ginger family, which is widely grown in southern and south western tropical Asia region.

Turmeric has got very important preventive and defensive properties against certain pathologies, as evidenced in scientific studies carried out in India, where turmeric is widely used by the population as a component of curry (*Kocaadam & Şanlier, Crit Rev Food Sci Nutr, 2017*).

The three main actions of turmeric pass through the contained substance curcumin:

- Antioxidant action and defense against free radicals. We must know that in producing energy our cells produce waste. Free radicals can be considered as waste products of energy production and, when in excess, they can damage cells and tissues in various ways.
- Anti-inflammatory action: curcumin has a direct action where there is localized inflammation. Some years ago some researchers at University of Bologna (Italy) proposed the term Inflammaging, indicating how the excessive inflammation is important in triggering the process of aging. Considering this, turmeric can be really considered an anti-aging food!
- Purifying action: curcumin helps the liver to dispose of exogenous substances.

DID YOU KNOW that turmeric and black pepper are good friends? The main bioactive substance of turmeric is curcumin. Curcumin is a incredibly powerful antioxidant (its antioxidant power is estimated to be about 300 times stronger than vitamin E!) with anti-inflammatory, antiviral, hepatoprotective, hypertensive, cholesterol lowering activities. Piperine, the molecule responsible for the pungency of black pepper, is able to increase the bioavailability of curcumin, namely the absorption and the entry of curcumin in our body. Therefore when you are employing turmeric in your dishes, ensure a splash of black pepper to increase the benefits of curcumin!

Walnuts: a treasure inside a shell

Juglans regia

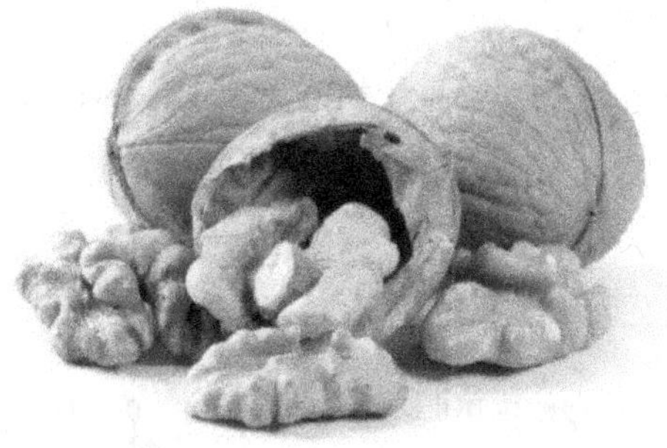

Walnuts are very important delights for their nutritional contributions that should never be missing in our recipes. Let's take a look to the elaborate anatomy of its fruit: the fruit is made up of an outer green shell cover (or husk), the middle shell which must be cracked to release the kernel, a thin layer known as skin (or the seed coat), and finally, the kernel. The nutritional importance of walnut fruit is ascribed to its kernel, which is the edible part.

The delicious kernel has multiple nutritional properties: rich in proteins, vitamins, minerals, fibers, and unsaturated and polyunsaturated fats. Noteworthy, they are rich in alpha-Linolenic acid, an omega-3 polyunsaturated fatty acid. Omega-3 fatty acids are associated to a number of healthy effects ranging from cardiovascular and heart protection, brain function, eye health and anti-inflammatory effects. Taking in account that omega-3 fatty acids are termed essential fats, as the body is not able to synthetize them and must take them through food and that western diet is, unfortunately, low in omega-3 fats, find a way to get enough walnuts intake in your diet! Excellent source of omega-3 fatty acids is fish, especially blue fish.

Regarding polyphenols, walnuts are one of the most important sources of total polyphenols among common foods, with a reported content of up to 2,5g per 100 g. One of the most abundant polyphenol is ellagitannin, associated to reduction of adiposity, LDL-cholesterol (the "bad" one) and glycemia (*Ros et al., Curr Opin Clin Nutr Metab Care, 2018*).

Among SIRT1-activating molecules, the most prominent in walnuts is gallic acid, a phenolic acid (*Jahanban-Esfahlan et al., Molecules, 2019*).

Walnuts are also rich in phytosterols, nutrients with cholesterol-lowering effect.

How Does The Sirtfood Diet Work?

The Sirtfood Diet is on everyone's lips right now. This is because, unlike most diets, it allows foods like chocolate and red wine: so good news for gourmets who want to slim by indulging in small pleasures!

Your goal will be to consume as many foods as possible from the Sirt Foods category to activate sirtuins in the body.

The Sirtfood diet has two phases that last a total of three weeks: one for weight loss or slimming, one for maintenance, which both lasts a total of 3 weeks.

Phase 1: Slimming

The first phase (the slimming phase) lasts one week and involves moderate caloric restriction and lots of green juice, a powerful tool that we will introduce soon. It is intended to boost your weight loss and help you lose until 7 pounds (3 kg) in seven days. The week is in turn, divided into two sub-phases and represents the most difficult part of the diet to overcome since few calories can be consumed, and there are few dietary variations. However after this challenging part, the road is downhill and you can start enjoying the pleasure of a diet that does not "remove" but does "add". During the first 3 days of the first phase, calorie intake is limited to 1,000 calories. You drink three green juices a day plus a meal (usually the lunch). Be sure to fill your meal with Sirt Food to take advantage of all their polyphenols.

For the remaining 4 days of the week, the calories go from 1,000 to 1,500 and two solid meals and two green juices are taken.

This is the phase during which the loss of the first 3 kg should occur.

Phase 2: Maintenance

The second phase is the maintenance phase. It lasts two weeks and helps you to consolidate the sacrifices made during the first phase of weight loss. In this phase, it is no longer useful to count calories, as there is no specific calorie limit. Instead, you eat three meals full of Sirt Foods and one green juice a day.

The Green Juice

The green juice is a very powerful friend for people undergoing to Sirtfood diet. In order to speed up the melting of fat induced by SIRT1 and, consequently, the weight loss, it is necessary to consume the maximum of foods that contain polyphenols able to activate SIRT1 and other sirtuins, namely the Sirt Foods we have seen previously.

With so many fruits and vegetables among Sirt Foods, it is possible to prepare the green juices to make the diet even more "soft" and fresh. The green juice take a crucial part in the diet and it is important that you learn how to make it during the days. Do not be scared, the method is very simple. You will need a juicer centrifuge or a blender and a kitchen scale, as the ingredients are listed by weight. The recipe is the following:

Ingredients:

- 75 grams (2.5 oz) kale

- 30 grams (1 oz) arugula (arugula)

- 5 grams (a handful) of parsley

- 5 grams (a handful) of lovage (optional)

- Two 2-3 celery stalks (leaves included)

- 1 cm (0.5 in) ginger

- Half a green apple

- Half a lemon

- Half a teaspoon of matcha green tea

Mix all the ingredients, except the powdered green tea and lemon, and pour them into a glass. Juice the lemon by hand, then mix the lemon juice and green tea powder in your juice mixing well everything.

The green juice is now ready to be enjoyed, to fill your day with energy and to activate SIRT1 into your cells!

Thanks to the green juice composed of these Sirt fruits and vegetables rich in polyphenols, you will be able thanks to this component to fill you up with energy!

These juices will be not only tasty and rich in vitamins, SIRT1-activating polyphenols and other important nutrients but also excellent for your health! This drink is rich in antioxidants too and it is full of minerals, such as calcium, magnesium and iron. These elements strengthen the immune defenses, as well as the tissues of your body.

Regular consumption of green juices also helps prevent cardiovascular disease.

The energy contained in green juices will help to assimilate enzymes, which are precious allies for digestion.

It is also very useful in removing toxins and natural waste from your body.

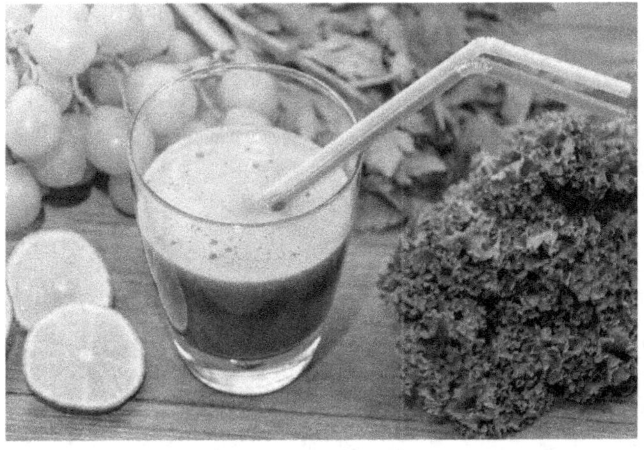

The Green Juice

After The Diet

You can repeat these two phases as often as you like for additional weight loss. However, it is encouraging to continue to "*sirtify*" your diet after completing these phases by regularly incorporating Sirt Foods into your meals. You can also include Sirt Foods in your diet as a snack or in recipes you already use. It is encouraged to continue drinking green juice every day. In this way, the Sirtfood diet becomes more of a lifestyle change than a single diet.

A Lifestyle Change for a Full Life

The Sirtfood Diet is arguably the only diet in the world to encourage consumption of chocolate and red wine. Too good to be true, and yet!

By favoring Sirt Foods consumption, this diet aims to improve your mode of feeding yourself. This diet really want to help you to make the definitive shift between "eating for feeding" to "eating for nourishing yourself". Trust me, this is really the paradigm shift that you need to change your life quality. It is not a matter of lose weight or reduce the fatty belly! Rather, it is first of all a matter of eating healthy for a full and joyful life. If you start eating Sirt Foods, maybe at the beginning you will miss the hamburgers, the French fries, the sugar-filled soft drinks and the donuts. However after including more and more good and healthy Sirt Foods, you will start to feel again the energy to face up your days, and you will feel that cooking and eating Sirt foods give you much more pleasure and satisfaction than filling your stomach with a supersize hamburger with French fries! At the end you won't have anymore the desire of eating junk food because you will have understood that eating Sirt Food you live much better.

We have seen that among this gourmet "elected" Sirt Foods there are many fruits and vegetables such as apples, fruits, strawberries, kale but also parsley, red onion, capers, green tea, soy, turmeric, olive oil, coffee and, more surprisingly, red wine and chocolate (dark of course)! For the most suspicious, know that the countries where people eat mostly exactly these food are among the world's healthiest populations.

This diet is really a good help to lose weight without starving yourself, even by consuming foods that are often prohibited in other diets. Forget the old-fashioned "low caloric" or "only green vegetable" or "zero-carb" diets!

Fibers: Sirt Foods extra benefits

As you probably noted, many of the Sirt Foods presented are either fruits or vegetables. This gives you an extra advantage when you eat them. Indeed, fruits and vegetables are the best sources of fibers we have at disposal.

Fibers are defined as non-nutrients: in fact, they do not provide energy to our body, nor they possess vitamin-like activity.

So why are they so important for our organism?

The answer relies mainly in our gut.

The intestine is a crucial organ for the absorption of nutrients and water coming from diet. However, there is much more to say. In the intestine resides the so-called intestinal microbiota. Also known (incorrectly) as intestinal microflora, the intestinal microbiota is the collection of all the species of microorganisms that live in our intestine. Their number is huge! The microorganisms inhabiting the gastro-intestinal tract has been estimated to exceed 10^{14} (i.e. 100.000.000.000.000 microorganisms!). The bacterial cells encompasses the number of human cells in all our body of about 10 times!

The microbiota offers us many benefits, through a range of physiological functions: it strengthens gut integrity, protects against pathogens and regulates host immunity (*Thursby & Juge, Biochem J, 2017*). However, these mechanisms can be disrupted if microbial composition is altered, in a pro-pathologic condition known as dysbiosis. Excess of sugar and saturated fats in the diet, alcohol, smoking, antibiotics and other factors are common cause of dysbiosis. Several line of recent evidence are pointing toward an increasingly important role of microbiota in our health, not only for the gut, but for all our body.

In this context, fibers are precious allies to prevent dysbiosis and to maintain intestinal microbiota integrity. However, not all fibers are the same: a useful classification distinguishes fibers among soluble and insoluble fibers.

Soluble fibers absorb water, are resistant to digestion in the upper part of the intestine and are fermented, at least partly, by the intestinal microbiota. Using soluble fibers as a source of energy for themselves, bacteria of microbiota proliferate and grow, allowing us to benefit from all their protective activities. For this reason, soluble fibers can also be referred with the name of "prebiotics" (maybe you have already heard of this term), as they stimulate the health and the proliferation of our good microbiota. Thanks to the absorption of water and the formation of a viscous gel, soluble fibers can also help control blood cholesterol levels and reduce the absorption of sugars introduced in the diet.

The second type of fibers are called insoluble fibers. They have the ability to absorb little water and are used only in a very small part by the intestinal microbiota. They therefore promote an increase in the volume of feces with the consequent increase in the speed of intestinal transit. This is very important, as in this way there is a continuous flux along the intestine, without stagnation and accumulation of potentially harmful substances in the lumen of the gut. Insoluble fibers are good friends against constipation and for a healthy intestinal regularity.

The benefits of fiber do not end there! Indeed, including fiber regularly in the diet ensures proper blood glucose (glycemia) control and prevent hyperglycemia occurrence. As we previously mentioned, steady hyperglycemia is one of the first steps that leads to insulin resistance and to diabetes. Eating a meal containing mainly carbohydrates means that our digestive tract rapidly break up (digest) the carbohydrates in smallest pieces, usually glucose, so that all the glucose molecules are very rapidly freed and ready to enter the blood all together leading to hyperglycemia. But if we eat a meal containing at the same time carbohydrates together with fibers, we help to attenuates the speed of entry of glucose (derived from carbohydrates) from lumen of intestine to the blood. In simply words, our digestive enzymes "lose time" trying to digest fibers (actually they are composed of carbon hydrogen and oxygen just like carbohydrates, but they are not digestible) and this slows down digestion of carbohydrates. Moreover, fibers increase the volume of material that reaches the intestine, creating a structure that makes it slower for digestive enzymes to find carbohydrates to break down.

In conclusion, fibers are really friend of your diet and Sirt foods are plenty of fibers. Be sure fibers are always present in your meals. Besides fueling you meals with vegetables, another good idea is choosing whole grains rather food made with refined flour. The former contain the fibers of the plant of origin, as well as vitamins and minerals, the latter is emptied of all the nutrients, fibers included.

Vitamin B3: a crucial tool for SIRT1 activity

I have always tried to not stuff this book with scientific terms, if not necessary. However, in this case I must go a little bit deeper in technical language to explain why specific vitamin, vitamin B3, is so important for SIRT1 activity.

Well, we have previously seen that SIRT1 is, biochemically speaking, an enzyme, more precisely a NAD-dependent deacetylase. This means that its specific function is to remove a sort of "tag" from other proteins. The tag is an "acetyle group", from which the name "deacetylase", but this is not particularly important for us now. What is worth of our attention is that "NAD-dependent" in the name: this implies that SIRT1 is an enzyme that works in dependence of the so-called NAD.

Who is NAD?

Well, NAD (or Nicotinamide Adenine Dinucleotide) is a cofactor (or coenzyme) that is central to our metabolism. It is present in all human cells, and it helps the functions of many enzymes and participates to carbohydrates and fat metabolism.

To better understand its importance, let's make this example: think to SIRT1 as a fisherman. To properly do his job, the fisherman must have a fisher pole. Obviously the fisher pole is completely useless alone. However, the activity of the fisherman is much more effective if he employs the fisher pole when going fishing! So, that's it: SIRT1 is the fisherman who perform the activity, while NAD is the fisher pole, a crucial tool for SIRT1 activity.

Therefore, NAD is very important for Sirtfood Diet, and having enough quantity in the body is crucial to make sure SIRT1 activity goes at 100% of its performance.

You can ask how to make enough NAD or where we can find NAD in the food. Actually, the best way to have proper amount of NAD in the body is to assume enough quantity of vitamin B3 (or Niacin).

Vitamin B3 is indeed the precursor for NAD (the body use vitamin B3 to build new NAD molecules). As the name says (in ancient Latin "vita" means "life") vitamin B3 is a very important nutrient for our health. The human body is not able to synthetize it, so vitamin B3 must come from the diet, mainly from food of animal origin like meat and fish (eggs instead contain low amount vitamin B3).

It can be also found also in the vegetal kingdom: whole grains, spinach, nuts, and among the Sirt Foods coffee and chili peppers.

Deficiency of vitamin B3 can cause pellagra, a disease whose symptoms include inflamed skin, diarrhea, dementia, and sores in the mouth. Noteworthy, vitamin B3 can also be called vitamin PP (Pellagra Preventing).

Remember: not suffering of pellagra does not mean that you have optimal amount of vitamin B3 in your body.

SIRT1 and AMPK: the "hunger" brothers

To understand who AMPK, a good friend of SIRT1, is and why it is important in the Sirtfood diet, we must before understand what is ATP.

Maybe all of us have a vague memory of ATP from school. ATP (Adenosine triphosphate) is the exchange currency that body uses to carry out most of its biochemical reactions and therefore all its physiological functions. When you go outside for a walk or a run or just study or read this book, you have an energy expenditure and you use ATP to pay it. If the cells, especially in the skeletal muscle (for example after a workout at the gym), start running out of ATP, AMPK come in action!

AMPK (AMP-Activated Protein Kinase) is a protein, more precisely an enzyme (like SIRT1 is). AMPK is particularly abundant inside the cytoplasm of myocytes, in the skeletal muscle. It is present also in other kind of cells of our body, but this goes beyond the scope of this book. When ATP is going to be depleted in the cell, AMPK "awakens" and start to perform his job, which is very complicated. The scope of his job, however, is much easier to understand than the mechanism, and it is the following: AMPK prompt many biological processes aimed to replenish cellular ATP stocks. For example, AMPK stimulates the muscle cells to absorb glucose from the blood, which is employed to produce new ATP (new fuel). AMPK also stimulates fatty acid oxidation within mitochondria, the main ATP producers, and increases the number of mitochondria itself. Actually, the story is a little bit more complicated, but we can summarize everything saying that the main actions of AMPK are (1) the lowering of glycemia leading to a better insulin sensitivity, and (2) the burning of fats. Not bad!

Do you feel like having already heard of this story and these activities when we talked about the functions of SIRT1? Indeed SIRT1 and AMPK have many elements in common. I sometimes call them the two "hunger brothers", as both of their actions are activated in situations of deprivation: SIRT1 is activated by caloric restriction, AMPK by exhaustion of cellular ATP.

We can ask ourselves how to activate AMPK, in other words how to deplete ATP in the myocytes. Well, as for SIRT1, a good method is training hard or undergoing caloric restriction. Not always easy. Of course, a good strategy plan to optimize our body composition should always consider a training plan with at least 2-3 training a week but, as already mentioned, long caloric restriction is not always possible and/or easy and/or advisable.

The nice thing (one of the many nice thing) of Sirtfood diet is that it activates AMPK in the same way it activates SIRT1, without starving and without training hard like an Olympic athlete. How? Still with polyphenols which activate SIRT1. Resveratrol is, in particular, a good and well recognized AMPK activator, as well as SIRT1 activator. In the 2011 study of Timmers and colleagues performed in obese human we have previously seen, the supplementation of resveratrol markedly activated AMPK too, not only SIRT1 (*Timmers et al., Cell Metab, 2011*).

There is more, not only resveratrol activates both SIRT1 and AMPK but, a cross-talk between SIRT1 and AMPK pathways occur in different types of tissues and cells. For example, in skeletal muscle AMPK enhances SIRT1 activity by increasing cellular NAD levels (*Wang et al., FEBS Lett, 2011*). Do you understand now why I call them the "hunger brothers"?

To date, the best science-based nutritional option we have at disposal to mimic caloric restriction is Sirtfood diet which, with its great supply of polyphenols is able to activate the two synergic pathways of SIRT1 and AMPK. For example, drinking during the day the green juice is very useful not only for its great polyphenols provision, but also because it is particularly rich of water and fibers. We all know that water is so important for our health. We are composed mostly of water (about 70% of you and me is made of water!) and we can truly say water is the most important nutrient of our diet. We have also seen the importance of fibers previously. I want to make you note now that neither water nor fibers give energy to our body. ATP cannot be made neither from water nor from fibers. Thus, drinking the green juice helps you feel satiated and with the full stomach. At the same time it brings few calories and therefore allows a lower level of ATP in the cells with consequent greater activation of AMPK (in addition to SIRT1).

Conclusions

When I begun to write this book I had two main aims. The first one was to give a scientific opinion and, at the same time, an explanation of how these mechanisms worked. Secondly, I wanted to give to the reader some useful informations about the functioning of its body and to make him/her understand as best as possible how Sirtfoods diet works and the most interesting properties of Sirt Foods.

I decided to write this book as soon as I came across the book "Sirt Food Diet" of Aidan Goggins and Glen Matten. Once read it, I understood that the science behind this diet was very solid. Many of the molecular mechanisms underlying SIRT1 functioning in caloric restriction, its interplay with other molecular players (such as AMPK) and how to use resveratrol and other SIRT1-activating polyphenols as a switch to these processes are indeed well known. If you want to lose weight without suffering by depriving yourself of the pleasure of good genuine foods, the Sirtfood Diet is absolutely a suitable solution for you. By combining pleasure and simplicity, this slimming method promises to lose until 3 kg in the first week, a boon for those who want to lose weight quickly and healthy at the same time.

The first phase of seven days could be the most difficult part because, in the first three days, the daily calorie energy intake is limited to 1,000 calories and, in the next four days, we allow ourselves to be close to the 1,500 daily calories mark. However, once overcome this effort, you will feel energetic and you will not need any more to care about calories. So remember, it is just one week, not caloric restriction for life! Furthermore, the green juice will help greatly to "mask" the hunger effect of caloric restriction. In the second phase, which extends over fourteen days, you will eat three equilibrate meal, rich of Sirt Foods daily, and the green juice once. Mid-morning or mid-afternoon snacks are allowed, but assure to fill them of Sirt Foods. Unlike its peers, this weight loss program is not based solely on a diet composed of fruits and vegetables but also offers greater freedom in the choice of food by authorizing, for example, chocolate. Therefore, if you want lose weight and live a better quality life without suffering by depriving yourself of gourmet foods, the Sirtfood Diet is the most suitable solution. Of course remember that equilibrium is always important and that variety in nutrition is always needed (among Sirt Foods too). Nevertheless, the choices among Sirt Foods are many (more than twenty), thus you will be able to experiments different food and different food combinations and you will not have to eat always the same things. As mentioned before, Sirtfood diet is not a diet that exclude foods, rather it is a diet that add foods (and adds polyphenols). Therefore, if you are very fond with a particular food that does not belong to Sirt Foods, you can continue to eat it, just remember to "*sirtify*" your meals combining it with Sirt Foods.

Consequently, rather than subjecting the body to the stress of such a diet and its long-term effects, we can instead focus on its daily consumption of foods rich in sirtuins SIRT1-activating polyphenols.

The Sirtfood diet is a breakthrough balanced diet plan backed by scientific research. Being on it for two weeks will help you shed fat without causing muscle loss. We have seen the great importance of muscle mass to speed up our metabolism and to consume energy (and excessive fat) through its mitochondria. We have also seen the importance of fibers provided by Sirt Foods and that vitamin B3 is an important vitamin for the proper functioning of SIRT1 action. Of course, also other vitamins are fundamental for our body health too: the variety of foods we eat will allow us to have good stocks of all of them.

The Sirtfood diet has been criticized because many of the scientific results on which it is based come from studies carried out on model organisms, starting from our good friend *yeast Saccharomyces cerevisiae* up to mammals closer to us, like the mouse. Critics argue that the results obtained in model organisms may not necessarily hold true in humans.

Although I am not particularly in agreement with these criticisms (even if their initial assumption is correct), I believe it is important to mention them because they give further food for thought. In fact, an important consideration must be made: although, in theory, it is true that the results obtained in a model organism may not be similar in humans, it must be said that, as regards SIRT1 and other sirtuins of model organisms, this is very unlikely.

When we talk about SIRT1 and sirtuins, we talk about a group of very ancient proteins that are crucial for survival. Since the family of sirtuins is highly preserved among living organisms, the function of the various sirtuins is also preserved. So we can assume in a relatively safe way that most of the effects found in Sir2 (the sirtuin analog to SIRT1 of the yeast *Saccharomyces cerevisiae* we have previously seen) are also present in the human SIRT1. Science goes on and time will give more and more indications but I am confident of scientific goodness of Sirtfood diet. The same authors of the book "The Sirt diet" who have tested their diet with more than excellent results in human people give further support! Furthermore, many populations whose inhabitants have a very high health index and a high life expectancy have consumed many of the Sirt Foods for millennia. Isn't this a kind of large-scale scientific experiment?

With this, I think that you have all you need to have a good introduction to Sirtfood diet. But the road has just begun! Now you can start having fun in the kitchen (in the next pages I have left you some ideas of some of my favorite recipes so that you can gain practical confidence with all the Sirt Foods). In addition, and above all, you can really understand freely if this diet is for you or not with the knowledge I gave you in this book.

I strongly believe that it is much better for people to understand than to believe. Here I did not try to convince you that Sirtfood diet is good for you. Instead, I tried to make you understand how Sirtfood works. Understanding is the only way to be free; blindly believing is the way to slavery. Be always curious about things of life! Be curious about nutrition, which is source of life for our bodies! Time spent in learning is never lost!

Questions & Answers

Here find some of the most frequently asked questions about Sirtfood diet.

Is this diet useful only for losing weight?

No! Sirtfood diet is an optimal choice not only to lose weight but also to introduce foods and nutrients that activate SIRT1 and other sirtuins. These protein are super-regulators of our metabolism and they perform a number of activity with eventually results better health outcomes. Even if you are already in your optimal shape, you can benefit much from the healthy outcomes of Sirtfood diet.

Can I eat meat / fish / eggs on the Sirtfood diet?

Yes, you can eat animal proteins on the Sirtfood diet. As explained in the text, Sirtfood diet does not remove but it adds. The important thing is therefore that you include Sirt Foods into your diet. If you like meat you can include it in your diet. Fish and eggs are not only accepted, but it is invited to you that you eat them as they are wonderful source of high valuable proteins. Fish (especially blue fish and salmon) are great source of the essential fatty acids omega-3 and eggs are really good for your health.

Can I substitute buckwheat products with normal flour products?

You can if you really want, but is much better to include it in your choices among Sirt Foods. Not eating it means losing a good opportunity to absorb good SIRT1-activating polyphenols. Furthermore, buckwheat is a good source of fiber and vitamins and it has got a low glycemic index. White flour is, on the other hand, low in nutrients and it has a high glycemic index, meaning that it raises too much your glycemia after eating it.

Is Sirtfood diet gluten free?

All the Sirt Foods are naturally devoid of gluten, therefore Sirtfood diet is gluten free. If you must avoid gluten in your diet you can follow Sirtfood diet.

Is Sirtfood diet lactose free?

Sirt Foods are naturally devoid of lactose, therefore Sirtfood diet is perfectly suitable for those who are lactose intolerant.

Can I change the recipe of green juice?

Yes you can. Consider the Green Juice presented as a basis, a starting point. Then you can try to adjust the dosage of ingredients, depending to your tastes and you can also try to change the ingredients (remove/add something), in order to make the preparation of green juice more funny. In this way you will always feel like drinking something new and you will never be tired of drinking the same juice. Every day can be different!

I am pregnant. Can I follow Sirtfood diet ?

It is better to not follow as the first part of the diet (phase 1) include a caloric restriction. You can anyway *sirtify* your diet by introducing Sirt Foods in your normal diet. Be cautious with caffeine-containing foods (coffee and matcha tea) and red wine (alcohol should be completely avoid during pregnancy but you can use it for cooking: with the heat alcohol evaporates and goes away). Anyway, I suggest you to consult your doctor before change your diet style during pregnancy.

Is Sirtfood diet suitable for children?

Sirtfood diet is not suitable for children as the first part of the diet (phase 1) include a caloric restriction. However children favorite recipes can be *sirtified* in order to make them benefit to the Sirt Food positive effects on health! Of course, coffee and matcha tea (due to the presence of caffeine) and red wine (due to the presence of alcohol) should not be given to children at all.

Must I follow phase 1 for 7 days or also 1-2 days less are ok?

Sirtfood is elastic, it is not a "follow-this-rule!" diet. If you feel you are not able to follow entirely the phase 1, you can reduce the days in which you undergo to phase 1. You will still benefit from it.

I assume drugs. Can I follow Sirtfood diets?

If you are assuming drugs it is better to consult your doctor before starting following Sirtfood diet.

How many times can I repeat phase 1 + phase 2?

You can repeat phase 1 + phase 2 how many times you want, in order to always have a high level of activation of SIRT1 and other sirtuins.

Recipes

My supervisor professor during my PhD years told me once that a good biologist should be also a good chef. I agreed with him. I've always considered a kitchen like a laboratory. However, in the kitchen experiments are much more delicious and good to eat! I believe that a good chef should be also a scientist too. A good secret to excel in cooking is also trying new things and learning from your mistakes with scientific mind and improving your recipes as if they were laboratory experiments.

In the following recipes (which are by no means exhaustive) I want to give you some ideas to test yourself in many way to employ Sirt Foods in your kitchen. Remember that the ingredients amounts indicated are a sort of starting point from which you can then experiment and try, releasing your creativity. Indeed many of the recipes and the quantities of ingredients can be varied according to your taste.

Moreover, I tried my best to include recipes that would be easy and quick to do, in order to be followed by everyone. You won't need to do a master's in *haute cuisine*!

The following are my favorite Sirt recipes. There are many others, but these are the ones I most frequently do on my own. I roughly divided them in sweet recipes and salty recipes.

Sweet Recipes

Greek Yogurt Bowl with Strawberries and Walnuts

This recipe is for 1 person and take less than 5 minutes to be prepared.

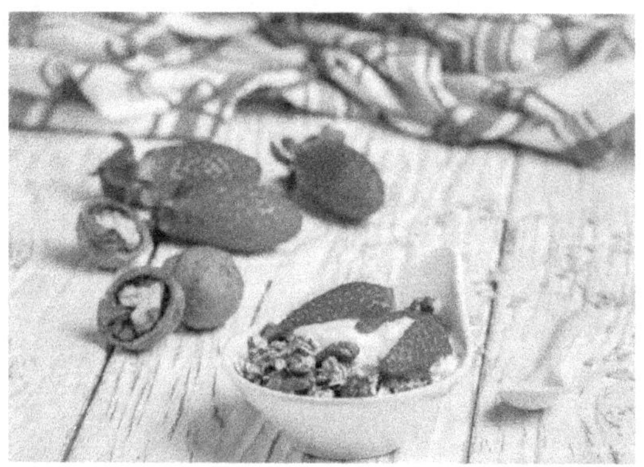

Ingredients:

- 170 g plain yogurt;

- 40 g organic buckwheat flakes;

- 5-6 strawberries (depending from dimensions of them), hulled and chopped;

- 3 walnuts (about 15 g), chopped;

- 1-2 dark chocolate squares (*optional*) ;

- 1 tsp honey (*optional*).

-

Instructions:

➢ Put the Greek yogurt inside a bowl.

➢ Add the buckwheat flakes and mix.

➢ Add the walnuts and the cleaned and chopped strawberries.

➢ If you wish, decorate your bowl with honey and/or dark chocolate squares broken into little pieces to make irresistible your bowl.

➢ Enjoy your breakfast (or snack) with a cup of coffee (or matcha tea) apart.

Wild fruits oat baskets

The amounts of ingredients are enough for 4 people. Time of preparation: 10-15 minutes. Baking time: 15 minutes.

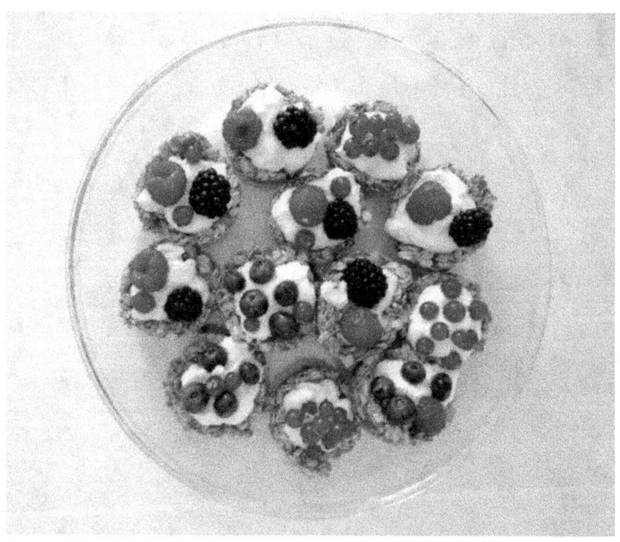

Ingredients:

- 110 g oat flakes;
- 100 g Medjoul dates, pitted;
- 60 g honey;

- 180 g Greek yogurt (0% fats);

- Wild fruits (just enough);

- 1 tbsp extra virgin olive oil;

- A pinch of cinnamon (*optional*).

Instructions:

➢ Pour the pitted dates in a mixer and blend them until you get a cream.

➢ Add the honey and, if you like, also the pinch of cinnamon.

➢ Mix all together and as soon the mixture is uniform add the oat flakes.

➢ Mix everything with a spoon.

➢ Grease a muffin pan with EVO oil and transfer a spoon of the mixture into the muffin pan.

➢ Transfer a spoonful of the oatmeal mixture into the molds and, using the back of the spoon, create baskets forming a cavity in the center.

➢ Bake in a preheated static oven at 170°C for 15 minutes. Then take out the baskets and let them cool

➢ Once cooled fill the baskets with Greek yogurt and decorate with wild fruits.

Dates stuffed with Walnuts

Super quick recipe but super super-tasty and full of energy, perfect for a post workout when you go to the gym or outside for jogging. Time of preparation: only 5 minutes!

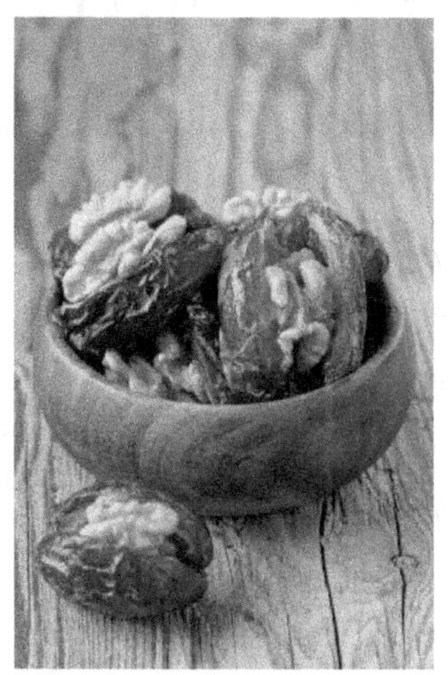

Ingredients:

- 100 g Medjoul dates, pitted;
- 4-5 walnuts (about 20 g), chopped;
- Greek yogurt (0% fats) (just enough) (*optional*).

Instructions:

- Cut the dates into two pieces and remove the core.
- If you wish, add the Greek yogurt inside the open date (*optional step*).
- Insert half a walnut kernel inside the open date.
- Enjoy!

Diced sweety apples

For 2 people. Time of preparation: 15 minutes

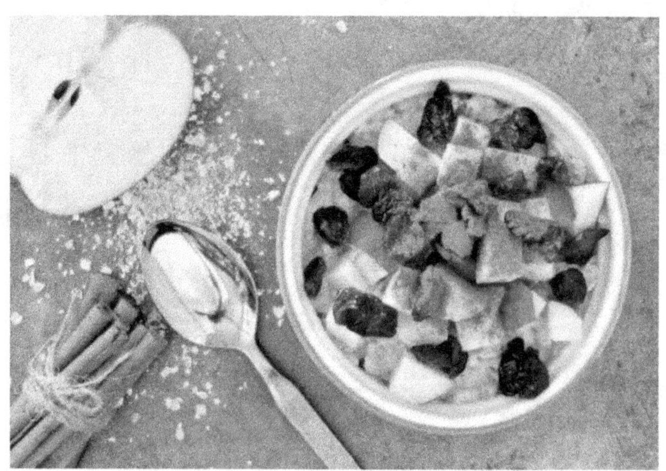

Ingredients:

- 2 red apples;

- Cocoa powder (just enough);

- 6 Medjoul dates, pitted;

- 1 tbsp brown sugar;

- A pinch of cinnamon (*optional*).

Instructions:

- ➢ Wash the apples and cut them into little cubes, keeping the peel.
- ➢ Add the apple cubes with brown sugar in a non-stick pan and heat for few minutes until the apple cubes soften.
- ➢ Pour in two bowls adding small pieces of dates, cocoa powder and cinnamon powder, according to your taste.

Salty Recipes

Arugula pesto

Although the procedure is very similar, the arugula pesto has a quite different taste than the classic "Genovese" pesto. Indeed, the arugula pesto has a stronger, slightly bitter taste. By changing the quantity of the ingredients you can also modulate the resulting flavor and after a few tests you can get the arugula pesto as good as you like.

Ingredients:

- 100 g arugula;
- 30 g pine nuts (if you do not find them you can opt for almonds);
- 1 clove of garlic;
- 80 g grated Parmesan;
- 100 mL extra virgin olive oil.

Instructions:

- ➢ Wash the rocket and dry it.

- Pour the rocket, pine nuts (or peeled almonds), grated Parmesan, garlic clove (deprived of the outer skin) and half of the EVO oil into a food processor. Blend at low speed and then add the remaining oil until creamy.
- The sauce obtained will be excellent as a sauce for pasta or on slices of grilled meat as well as in roasted bread as a snack.

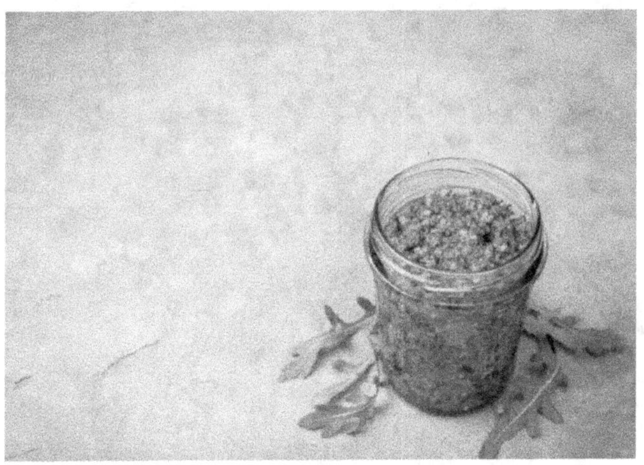

Spicy soba noodles

For 2 people. Time of preparation: 20 minutes

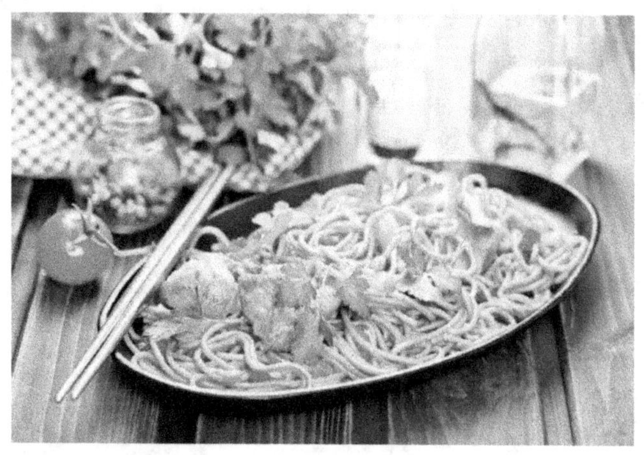

Ingredients:

- 160 soba noodles;
- Half red onion;
- 1 chilli pepper;
- 1 bell pepper;
- A pinch of turmeric;

- 1 handful parsley (alternatively you can use the same amount of lovage);
- 2 tbsp extra virgin olive oil;
- Soybean sprouts.

Instructions:

- ➢ Chop the onion and chili pepper and heat them in a non-stick pan with extra virgin olive oil.
- ➢ Cut the bell pepper into cubes and add it to the pan together with the mung bean sprouts. Cook for 10 minutes stirring occasionally and if necessary add a drop of water not to burn the vegetables.
- ➢ In the meantime, cook the soba noodles in a pot of boiling water following the directions on the package;
- ➢ Add the noodles to the pan and sauté over high heat for 1-2 minutes to flavor. With the heat off, add the turmeric and the chopped parsley (or lovage).
- ➢ Taste the freshly made spicy noodles.

DID YOU KNOW how capsaicin make your mouth **burn?** Eating chili peppers you feel fire and flames in your mouth. Noteworthy the temperature inside your mouth is not changed! What you feel is the activity of capsaicin molecule, which is able to activate thermo-receptors in the mouth as if there was hot in the mouth even if there is not! Capsaicin, in a sense, deceives our body. In response to this stress, the body causes a rapid release of adrenaline, giving a boost of energy to the body, activating the metabolism of fats, stimulating thermogenesis and supporting the basal metabolism. By virtue of these properties, capsaicin contained in chili peppers can help reduce body weight and has anti-obesity properties (*Zheng et al., Biosci Rep, 2017*).

Red Wine Chicken Strips

For 4 people. Time of preparation: 40-45 minutes

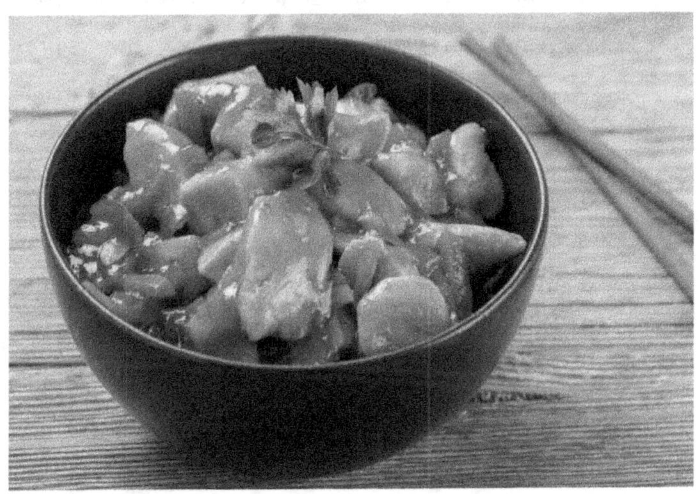

Ingredients:

- 1 Kg chicken breast;
- 2 glasses of red wine;
- 1 red onion;
- Half a rib of celery;
- 1 red bell pepper and 1 green bell pepper;

- Extra virgin olive oil (just enough);

- 1 tbsp soy sauce;

- Organic raw buckwheat.

Instructions:

- Cut the chicken breast into small pieces and place them in a bowl, add the red wine and the chopped chilli pepper and parsley, mix and leave marinating for at least 30 minutes.

- Meanwhile, chop the onion and celery and heat them in a non-stick pan with few drops of extra virgin olive oil. Add the two bell peppers cut into little sticks and cook for 10 minutes.

- Add the chicken, with the marinating liquid, into the pan and cook for about 15-20 minutes,

- Add soy sauce to give flavor.

- If you are hungry, serve with boiled rice or boiled buckwheat.

DID YOU KNOW all the colors of bell peppers? There are countless colors of peppers in the world: pink, purple, brown, orange, but the most common are yellow, red and green. Green peppers are nothing more than the immature version of yellow or red. As you can easily imagine, being an immature fruit, the green pepper is more bitter and has a fresher and more herbaceous flavor than the red ones ripened in the sun, sweeter and fruity. If green peppers are left to mature in the plant, the green color caused by the green molecule chlorophyll disappears and the brightest colors of carotenoids such as lutein and beta-carotene are left in place.

Sirt Salad

One of the best application of Sirt Foods are mixed salads. Actually, the Sirt Salad is not a true recipe, as it is simply a blend of different Sirt Foods (mostly vegetables) that you can mix together depending on your taste (and also on your fridge!). The union of this foods is not only a "panzer" of polyphenols, but also a synergy of flavors (any combination you experiment will always be new and savory!). Therefore, here I do not give you the amount of ingredients. Just make experiments and test your taste.

Ingredients for the base:

- Red chicory;
- Arugula;
- Celery.

Ingredients (for the optional additions):

- Capers;
- Soybean sprouts;
- Red onion;
- Walnuts;
- Apple in pieces;
- Parsley;

- Lovage.

Ingredients (for the seasoning):

- Extra virgin olive oil;

- A pinch of salt (*optional*);

- Black pepper (*optional*);

- Chili pepper (*optional*);

- Vinegar (the kind you prefer, *optional*)

Instructions:

- Cut the ingredients into pieces at the dimension you prefer;

- Put the ingredients you have chosen all together in a bowl;

- Season as you like (do not forget EVO oil!)

- Enjoy!

DID YOU KNOW that the belief that vegetables should be **used only as a side dish is wrong?** The vegetable must be, in terms of volume, the food most present in our diet at least in the main meals. The single dish should be divided in this way: 50% of the space to go to vegetables, 25% to whole grains and 25% to healthy proteins (such as lean meat, fish, eggs). Vegetables (especially Sirt vegetables) are an insurance for health and longevity. Season everything with the healthy and delicious extra virgin olive oil.

Kale chips

This recipe is very simple and very popular these days.

Do you want to eat delicious chips?

What if I offer you good and healthy at the same time? Well, get ready for the kale chips!

Ingredients:

- 400 g kale;
- 1 chilli pepper;
- A pinch of salt;
- 5 tbsp of extra virgin olive oil.

Instructions:

- Wash the kale leaves and dry them with paper towels or a dish towel.
- Cut the leaves into pieces and arrange them on the oven plate which you had covered with baking paper.
- Finely chop some chili pepper and mix it with extra virgin olive oil.

> Brush the pieces of curly kale leaves with the chili pepper flavored oil and cook them in the oven at 180°C for about 5-10 minutes, depending on your oven. Crispy chips will come out!

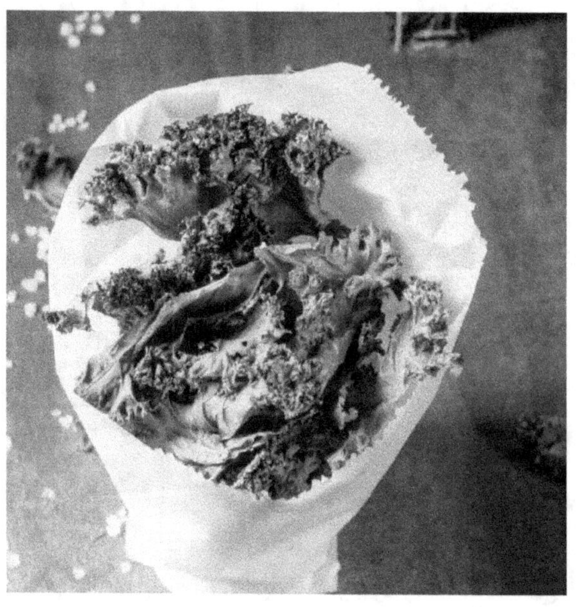

Sauteed Tofu with bell peppers

- 177 -

For 4 people. Time of preparation: 15 minutes. Time of cooking: 20 minutes

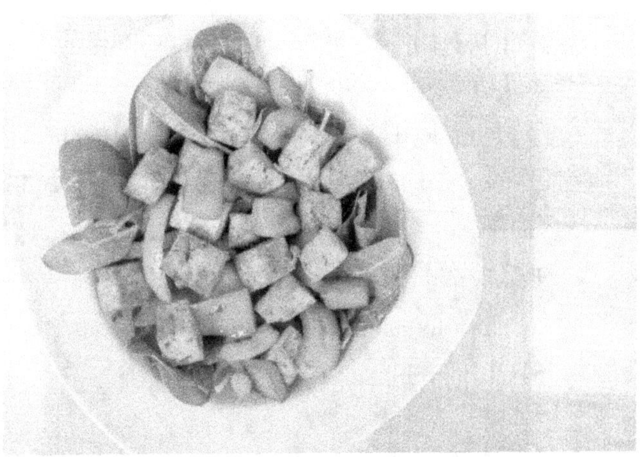

Ingredients:

- 300 g tofu;
- 1 bell pepper;
- Half red onion;
- 1 chili pepper;
- Soy sauce;

- Soybean sprouts

- Extra virgin olive oil;

- A handful of parsley.

Instructions:

➤ Wash and chop the red onion and heat it in a non-stick pan with 2 tablespoons of extra virgin olive oil and chopped chili pepper.

➤ Add the diced bell pepper and cook for 10 minutes.

➤ In the meantime, cut the tofu into cubes and add it to the pan. Cook it for about 5 minutes.

➤ Finally add the soybean sprouts and soy sauce and let flavor for a few minutes.

➤ Serve by sprinkling with chopped parsley.

DID YOU KNOW that bell peppers are wonderful **source of vitamin C?** We are used to associate vitamin C to lemons or oranges. However, according to United States Department of Agriculture (USDA) oranges contains about 59 mg of vitamin C per 100 g (skin excluded), while lemon contains about 53 mg of vitamin C per 100 g (skin excluded). If you eat a lemon (if you can!) you feel that it is more sour simply because it contains a higher amount of citric acid. As regards peppers, they contain 191 mg of vitamin C per 100 g!

Glossary

- 180 -

Adipocyte: Cell of the adipose tissue. It is specialized to synthetize and accumulate fats as an energy storage. It also synthetize and secretes hormones (for example adiponectin) that regulates metabolism.

Adiponectin: A hormone that is mainly secreted from the adipose tissue and combats obesity and diabetes, enhances insulin sensitivity, and promotes proper glucose homeostasis. Adiponectin can up-regulate SIRT1 and AMPK and thus promote metabolic fitness.

Adrenaline: Adrenaline, also known as epinephrine, is a hormone produced by the adrenal glands. It plays an important role in the "fight-or-flight" response by increasing blood flow to muscles, output of the heart and pupil dilation response. In adipose tissue it also increases lipolysis and release of fatty acids that can be in turn used as a source of energy by other organs (for example skeletal muscle).

Alkaloid: Organic substance containing nitrogen and produced in plants. Usually toxic for human bodies. Some alkaloids can be beneficial to human bodies at small quantities.

Amino Acid: A simple organic compound containing oxygen, hydrogen, carbon and nitrogen. It is the "brick" proteins are made of. In the human organism there are 20 different types of amino acid used to produce proteins. Different proteins are produced from different combination of the 20 amino acids.

AMPK: AMP-activated protein kinase. AMPK is an enzyme that plays a crucial role in cellular energy control and metabolism. It promotes glucose and fatty acids uptake and oxidation when cellular energy is low.

Antioxidant: A nutrient able to reduce damage of free radicals in the body, protecting cells and tissues. Antioxidants can be natural or artificial.

Apigenin: A polyphenol belonging to the flavonoid group. It is a yellow crystalline solid that has been used to dye wool. It is found in many fruits and vegetables, but parsley, celery and chamomile tea are the most common sources. It is a natural sirtuins activator.

Ascorbic Acid: Synonym of vitamin C.

ATP: Adenosine triphosphate. ATP is an organic compound which provides the energy needed for the many processes of living cells, e.g. muscle contraction, nerve impulse propagation, and synthesis of new molecules. It releases energy by the breaking of its molecular bonds. It is found in all known forms of life.

Butein: A natural molecule present in the plant kingdom. It activates sirtuins.

Caffeic Acid: A natural sirtuins activator. It is present in many different vegetal derived foods, such as coffee and dates.

Caffeine: Caffeine is a natural molecule belonging to methylxanthine class and found in many different plants. It is a strong central nervous system stimulant and it is the world's most widely consumed psychoactive drug. One of the most known and studied mechanism of action is the inhibition of specific receptors, called adenosine receptors, in the brain. By inhibiting adenosine receptors, caffeine induce awakeness and alert.

Caloric Restriction: A dietary regiment that provides ~70% of the calories of an ad libitum diet.

Capsaicin: Capsaicin is the active ingredient in chili peppers (Capsicum spp. plants). Present in the fruits (berries) and seeds of these plants. The violent and spicy flavor of the chili pepper, capable of enhancing a large number of dishes, is linked precisely to the abundant presence of Capsaicin.

Carbohydrate: A carbohydrate is a biomolecule consisting of carbon (C), hydrogen (H) and oxygen (O) atom. It is one of the three main macronutrients, along with proteins and fats. Carbohydrates can be divided in simple carbohydrates (or sugars), with a low molecular weight, and in complex carbohydrates, with a high molecular weight. Examples of sugars are glucose and sucrose (the cooking sugar); example of complex carbohydrate is amid. Carbohydrates consumed in food yield about 4 kilocalories of energy per gram.

Chlorogenic Acid: A polyphenol abundant in coffee. It is a natural sirtuins activator.

Cholesterol: Fat molecule with important structural functions in the cellular membranes. It is also the precursor of many important hormones (e.g. testosterone, estrogen). Excess of cholesterol in the body, especially in the forms LDL and VLDL are associated to cardio-vascular diseases.

Curcumin: A bright yellow phenolic compound that is the main constituent of turmeric powder, with many and diverse health-promoting effects, mainly anti-inflammatory, antioxidant and detoxifying.

Cytoplasm: The liquid content of the cell, excluding nucleus and other organelles.

Diabetes: A pathology in which the body's ability to produce or respond to the hormone insulin is impaired, resulting in abnormal metabolism of carbohydrates and elevated levels of glucose in the blood (hyperglycemia).

Daidzein: A polyphenol particularly abundant in soy and its derivatives, with cardiovascular protective effects.

DNA: Deoxyribonucleic acid. DNA is a biomolecule contained mainly in the nucleus. Its sequence codes the genetic information for all living beings.

Enzyme: An enzyme is a protein acting as a biological catalyst. A catalyst speed up chemical reactions.

Epicatechin: A polyphenol belonging to the flavonoid group. It is the most abundant polyphenol in cocoa. It is a natural sirtuins activator.

Epigallocatechin Gallate: (EGCG). The most important and abundant polyphenol in teas, particularly abundant in green tea and matcha tea. It is a natural sirtuins activator.

Epigenetics: Epigenetics is a branch of genetics that studies how DNA "expresses itself" in response to changes in the environment to which it is subject (e.g.: diet, physical activity, environmental or psychological stress, pollution, etc.).

Essential Amino Acids: An essential amino acid (or indispensable amino acid) is an amino acid that cannot be synthesized ex novo by the human body, and thus must be supplied in its diet.

Fat: Fats are one of the three main macronutrients, along with carbohydrates and proteins. Fat molecules consist of primarily carbon (C) and hydrogen (H) atoms and are insoluble in water (they are hydrophobic). Examples of fats include cholesterol, phospholipids, and triglycerides. Fats consumed in food yield about 9 kilocalories of energy per gram.

Fat Oxidation: Fat oxidation refers to the process of breaking down fatty acids. The process, which requires oxygen (from which the term "oxidation" comes from) consume fat, which is "burned" and produce ATP. Fat oxidation takes place in the mitochondria.

Fisetin: A plant polyphenol found in many plants, where it serves as a coloring agent (it confers yellow colour). It is also found in many fruits and vegetables, such as strawberries, apples, persimmons, onions, tea and cucumbers. It is a natural sirtuins activator.

Free Radicals: Unstable atoms and molecules able to damage cells, causing pathologies and aging. Main source of free radicals is the respiration taking place inside the mitochondria during cell respiration. In order to dispose of free radicals and to protect from diseases and aging, cells are provided of "shields" (such as the antioxidant molecules) able to inactivate excess of free radicals.

Gene: Physical and functional unit which contributes in the characterization of features passing from parents to offspring (e.g.: the color of the eyes). In other words a gene is a specific DNA sequence coding for an information. The expression of a gene allows for a specific activity of the organism. In other words, when a gene is activated, it produces a specific proteins that change somehow the activity of the cell and thus of the organism.

Genetics: Genetics is a branch of biology dealing with the study of genes, genetic variation, and heredity in organisms.

Genistein: A polyphenol particularly abundant in soy and its derivatives, with cardiovascular protective effects.

Genome: All the genetic informations (the genes) of an organism.

Glucose: The main sugar employed as a source of energy by human body and animals. Glucose is stored in animals as glycogen in muscle and liver and it is stored in plants as starch. Glucose is the starting material for producing ATP.

Glycemia: The amount of glucose in the blood. An unusually high concentration of glucose in the blood is termed "hyperglycemia", while an unusually low concentration of glucose in the blood is termed "Hypoglycemia". Causes of hyperglycemia is excessive consumption of carbohydrates, especially sugars.

Glycogen: Glycogen is a polysaccharide of glucose that serves as a form of energy storage in animals. In mammals glycogen is stored mainly in skeletal muscle and, secondly, in the liver. The amount of glycogen in the body is limited: around 500-800 g, even if it can vary much among individuals.

Guaranine: Synonym of caffeine.

HDL: High-density lipoprotein (HDL) is a complex of different molecules (mainly proteins and fats) which transport fat molecules around the body. Increasing concentrations of HDL particles are strongly associated with decreasing accumulation of atherosclerosis within the walls of arteries.

Hormone: Signaling molecule secreted in the blood from a cell. Carried by the blood, a hormone can reach many other different cells, communicating its signal and modifying the activity of these cells.

Hypothalamus: The hypothalamus is an area in the brain important for coordinating crucial mammalian physiological actions such as feeding, body temperature, energy expenditure and metabolism.

Inflammation: Part of the complex biological response of organism tissues to harmful stimuli, such as pathogens, or irritants. It is a physiologic activity of the organism; however, prolonged (chronic) inflammation is noxious and can lead to different pathologies.

Insulin: A little protein with acts as a hormone. It is secreted from pancreas and it helps to regulate the blood glucose level (glycemia) in animals by lowering glycemia when there is a condition of hyperglycemia.

Isoliquiritigenin: A polyphenol found in licorice and soy. It is a natural sirtuins activator.

Kaempferol: A polyphenol belonging to the flavonoid group. It is found in a variety of plants and plant-derived foods including kale, capers, arugula, beans, tea, spinach, broccoli and ginger. It is a natural sirtuins activator.

LDL: Low-density lipoprotein (LDL) is a complex of different molecules (mainly proteins and fats) which transport fat molecules around the body. Excess of LDL has been shown harmful as it can accumulate on lumen of arteries resulting in atherosclerosis.

Luteolin: A polyphenol belonging to the flavonoid group. Dietary sources include celery, broccoli, green pepper, parsley, olive oil, oranges. It is a natural sirtuins activator.

Meta-analysis: A meta-analysis is a statistical analysis that combines the results of multiple scientific studies, addressing the same question. It represents, among all the kind of publications in scientific literature, the one that gives the higher level of confidence and security about what it says.

Metabolism: All the biochemical reactions producing or consuming energy that take place in living beings.

Mitochondrion: Mitochondria are double-membrane-provided organelles found in cells of most eukaryotic organisms, including all mammals. All human cells are provided of mitochondria, excluding some exceptions (for example, mature mammalian red blood cells). The most prominent roles of mitochondria are to produce ATP the energy currency of the cell, through respiration, and to regulate cellular metabolism.

Myocyte: Muscle cell.

Myricetin: A polyphenol belonging to the flavonoid group. Common dietary sources include vegetables, citrus fruits, nuts, berries, tea, and red wine. It is a natural sirtuins activator.

NAD+: Nicotinamide adenine dinucleotide. One of the most important cofactors in living cells, it participates in many biochemical reaction of the metabolism, including the activity of SIRT1.

Nucleus: The nucleus is an organelle found inside animal and vegetal cells. It contains the majority of the cell's genetic material. This material is organized as DNA molecules.

Nutrient: A molecule found in food that our body employ to survive, grow and perform all its physiological activities.

Oleuropein: The main polyphenol present in olive oil and is the main nutrient responsible for the bitter taste of olives and its oil. It is a natural sirtuins activator.

PGC-1 alpha: Key regulator of energy metabolism. It stimulates the production of new mitochondria in the cells.

Piceatannol: A polyphenol abundant in red wine. In chemistry, it is considered as an analog of resveratrol as their chemical formula are similar. It is a natural sirtuins activator.

Polyphenols: Polyphenols make up a family of around 5000 natural organic molecules found in the plant kingdom. As the name indicates, they are characterized by the presence of multiple phenolic groups associated in more or less complex structures. Polyphenols are natural antioxidants.

PPAR-gamma: Peroxisome proliferator-activated receptor gamma. Key regulator of energy metabolism. It stimulates synthesis and storage of fats.

Protein: Molecule constituted of one or more filaments of amino acids. Proteins are one of the three main macronutrients, along with fats and carbohydrates. Proteins consumed in food yields about 4 kilocalories of energy per gram.

Quercetin: A polyphenol belonging to the flavonoid group. It is particularly abundant in red onions, green tea, red wine, apples, wild berries, buckwheat, beans, lovage, capers, and kale. It is a natural sirtuins activator.

Resveratrol: The main polyphenol compound found in red wine and other plants. It has strong antioxidant properties. In nature, plants produce resveratrol to protect themselves from bacteria and parasites. It is a natural sirtuins activator. Besides red grapes, resveratrol is abundant also in blueberries and other wild berries and cocoa powder.

Rutin: Rutin is a composite molecule: it is made up of a polyphenolic part (quercetin) linked to a carbohydrate (rutinose). Rutin is particularly abundant in buckwheat, as well as in Citrus fruits, red wine and peppermint. Although not an essential compound for humans, it can be called "vitamin P". It is a natural sirtuins activator.

Sirt Food: A food highly enriched with specific polyphenols able to activate sirtuins.

SIRT1: (Silent information regulator T1). The most studied gene belonging to Sirtuins family and the most related to weight loss. It has been associated with a number of health-promoting functions in the organism.

Sirtuins: A class of genes that code for a class of enzymatic activity proteins. In humans there are 7 distinct sirtuins (SIRT1, SIRT2, ..., SIRT7). Sirtuins are important regulators of metabolism and mediate phenomena such as aging and resistance to stress. Caloric restriction, physical activity or Sirt Foods activate them.

Skeletal Muscle: Skeletal muscle is one of three major muscle types, the others being cardiac muscle and smooth muscle. Its main function is the movement of the body. It is under the voluntary control of the nervous system. Most of the skeletal muscles are linked to bones by bundles of collagen fibers known as tendons. There are around 640 skeletal muscles within the human body.

Starch: White substance occurring widely in plant tissues and obtained chiefly from cereals and potatoes. In plants, it is a polysaccharide of glucose, which functions as a carbohydrate store and is an important constituent of the human diet.

Theine: Synonym of caffeine.

Theobromine: Theobromine is a natural substance, abundant in cocoa. It is endowed with a mild diuretic, cardiotonic and vasodilatory action, especially at the coronary level. It belongs, like caffeine, to the family of alkaloids. However, unlike caffeine, theobromine has only a mild excitatory effect in the brain, estimated 10 times lower than the caffeine.

Vitamin C: Also known as ascorbic acid. It is one of the most important vitamins in our body. It is essential for the production of collagen, the most abundant protein of our body and it is one of the most abundant and important antioxidant molecule in the human body. It is a cofactor for the activity of many enzymes.

Bibliography

Alhowiriny, T. A., Al-rehaily, A. J., Tahir, K. E. H. El, Al-taweel, A. M., & Perveen, S. (2013). Molecular mechanisms that underlie the sexual stimulant actions of ginger (Zingiber officinale Rosocoe) and garden rocket (Eruca sativa L.). *Journal of Medicinal Plants Research, 7*(32), 2370–2379. https://doi.org/10.5897/JMPR12.821

Chang, H.-C., & Guarente, L. (2014). SIRT1 and other sirtuins in metabolism. *Trends in Endocrinology and Metabolism: TEM, 25*(3), 138–145. https://doi.org/10.1016/j.tem.2013.12.001

D'Antona, G., Ragni, M., Cardile, A., Tedesco, L., Dossena, M., Bruttini, F., … Nisoli, E. (2010). Branched-chain amino acid supplementation promotes survival and supports cardiac and skeletal muscle mitochondrial biogenesis in middle-aged mice. *Cell Metabolism, 12*(4), 362–372. https://doi.org/10.1016/j.cmet.2010.08.016

Ellam, S., & Williamson, G. (2013). Cocoa and human health. *Annual Review of Nutrition, 33*, 105–128. https://doi.org/10.1146/annurev-nutr-071811-150642

Farzaei, M. H., Abbasabadi, Z., Ardekani, M. R. S., Rahimi, R., & Farzaei, F. (2013). Parsley: a review of ethnopharmacology, phytochemistry and biological activities. *Journal of Traditional Chinese Medicine = Chung i Tsa Chih Ying Wen Pan, 33*(6), 815–826. https://doi.org/10.1016/s0254-6272(14)60018-2

Garrido-Bañuelos, G., Buica, A., Schückel, J., Zietsman, A. J. J., Willats, W. G. T., Moore, J. P., & Du Toit, W. J. (2019). Investigating the relationship between cell wall polysaccharide composition and the extractability of grape phenolic compounds into Shiraz wines. Part II: Extractability during fermentation into wines made from grapes of different ripeness levels. *Food Chemistry, 278*, 26–35. https://doi.org/10.1016/j.foodchem.2018.10.136

Giampieri, F., Forbes-Hernandez, T. Y., Gasparrini, M., Alvarez-Suarez, J. M., Afrin, S., Bompadre, S., … Battino, M. (2015). Strawberry as a health promoter:

an evidence based review. *Food & Function, 6*(5),
1386-1398. https://doi.org/10.1039/c5fo00147a

Goggins, A., Matten, G. (2016). The Sirt Food Diet.
Yellow Kite.

Goldstein, E. R., Ziegenfuss, T., Kalman, D., Kreider, R.,
Campbell, B., Wilborn, C., ... Antonio, J. (2010).
International society of sports nutrition position
stand: caffeine and performance. *Journal of the
International Society of Sports Nutrition, 7*(1), 5.
https://doi.org/10.1186/1550-2783-7-5

Heimler, D., Isolani, L., Vignolini, P., Tombelli, S., &
Romani, A. (2007). Polyphenol content and
antioxidative activity in some species of freshly
consumed salads. *Journal of Agricultural and Food
Chemistry, 55*(5), 1724-1729.
https://doi.org/10.1021/jf0628983

Howitz, K. T., Bitterman, K. J., Cohen, H. Y., Lamming,
D. W., Lavu, S., Wood, J. G., ... Sinclair, D. A.
(2003). Small molecule activators of sirtuins extend
Saccharomyces cerevisiae lifespan. *Nature,*

425(6954), 191–196.
https://doi.org/10.1038/nature01960

Imai, S.-I. (2009). The NAD World: a new systemic regulatory network for metabolism and aging--Sirt1, systemic NAD biosynthesis, and their importance. *Cell Biochemistry and Biophysics, 53*(2), 65–74. https://doi.org/10.1007/s12013-008-9041-4

Jahanban-Esfahlan, A., Ostadrahimi, A., Tabibiazar, M., & Amarowicz, R. (2019). A Comparative Review on the Extraction, Antioxidant Content and Antioxidant Potential of Different Parts of Walnut (Juglans regia L.) Fruit and Tree. *Molecules, 24*(11). https://doi.org/10.3390/molecules24112133

Kaeberlein, M., McVey, M., & Guarente, L. (1999). The SIR2/3/4 complex and SIR2 alone promote longevity in Saccharomyces cerevisiae by two different mechanisms. *Genes and Development, 13*(19), 2570–2580. https://doi.org/10.1101/gad.13.19.2570

Katz, D. L., Doughty, K., & Ali, A. (2011). Cocoa and Chocolate in Human Health and Disease.

ANTIOXIDANTS & REDOX SIGNALING,
15(10). https://doi.org/10.1089/ars.2010.3697

Kocaadam, B., & Şanlier, N. (2017). Curcumin, an active
component of turmeric (Curcuma longa), and its
effects on health. *Critical Reviews in Food Science
and Nutrition, 57*(13), 2889–2895.
https://doi.org/10.1080/10408398.2015.1077195

Kreft, S., Strukelj, B., Gaberscik, A., & Kreft, I. (2002).
Rutin in buckwheat herbs grown at different UV-B
radiation levels: comparison of two UV
spectrophotometric and an HPLC method. *Journal
of Experimental Botany, 53*(375), 1801–1804.
https://doi.org/10.1093/jxb/erf032

Kschonsek, J., Wolfram, T., Stöckl, A., & Böhm, V.
(2018). Polyphenolic Compounds Analysis of Old
and New Apple Cultivars and Contribution
of Polyphenolic Profile to the In Vitro Antioxidant
Capacity. *Antioxidants (Basel, Switzerland), 7*(1).
https://doi.org/10.3390/antiox7010020

Ma, L., Liu, G., Ding, M., Zong, G., Hu, F. B., Willett, W.
C., ... Sun, Q. (2020). Isoflavone intake and the risk

of coronary heart disease in US men and women: Results from 3 prospective cohort studies. *Circulation*, 1127–1137. https://doi.org/10.1161/CIRCULATIONAHA.119.041306

Picard, F., Kurtev, M., Chung, N., Topark-Ngarm, A., Senawong, T., Machado De Oliveira, R., ... Guarente, L. (2004). Sirt1 promotes fat mobilization in white adipocytes by repressing PPAR-gamma. *Nature, 429*(6993), 771–776. https://doi.org/10.1038/nature02583

Poole, R., Kennedy, O. J., Roderick, P., Fallowfield, J. A., Hayes, P. C., & Parkes, J. (2017). Coffee consumption and health: umbrella review of meta-analyses of multiple health outcomes. *BMJ (Clinical Research Ed.), 359*, j5024. https://doi.org/10.1136/bmj.j5024

Ros, E., Izquierdo-Pulido, M., & Sala-Vila, A. (2018). Beneficial effects of walnut consumption on human health: role of micronutrients. *Current Opinion in Clinical Nutrition and Metabolic Care, 21*(6), 498–

504.
https://doi.org/10.1097/MCO.0000000000000508

Salomón-Torres, R., Ortiz-Uribe, N., Valdez-Salas, B.,
Rosas-González, N., García-González, C., Chávez,
D., ... Krueger, R. (2019). Nutritional assessment,
phytochemical composition and antioxidant analysis
of the pulp and seed of medjool date grown in
Mexico. *PeerJ*, *7*, e6821.
https://doi.org/10.7717/peerj.6821

Satoh, A., Brace, C. S., Ben-Josef, G., West, T., Wozniak,
D. F., Holtzman, D. M., ... Imai, S. I. (2010). SIRT1
promotes the central adaptive response to diet
restriction through activation of the dorsomedial and
lateral nuclei of the hypothalamus. *Journal of
Neuroscience, 30*(30), 10220–10232.
https://doi.org/10.1523/JNEUROSCI.1385-10.2010

Sinclair, D. A. (2005). Toward a unified theory of caloric
restriction and longevity regulation. *Mechanisms of
Ageing and Development, 126*(9 SPEC. ISS.), 987–
1002. https://doi.org/10.1016/j.mad.2005.03.019

Thursby, E., & Juge, N. (2017). Introduction to the human gut microbiota. *The Biochemical Journal, 474*(11), 1823–1836. https://doi.org/10.1042/BCJ20160510

Timmers, S., Konings, E., Bilet, L., Houtkooper, R. H., van de Weijer, T., Goossens, G. H., … Schrauwen, P. (2011). Calorie restriction-like effects of 30 days of resveratrol supplementation on energy metabolism and metabolic profile in obese humans. *Cell Metabolism, 14*(5), 612–622. https://doi.org/10.1016/j.cmet.2011.10.002

Tsai, K.-L., Hung, C.-H., Chan, S.-H., Hsieh, P.-L., Ou, H.-C., Cheng, Y.-H., & Chu, P.-M. (2018). Chlorogenic Acid Protects Against oxLDL-Induced Oxidative Damage and Mitochondrial Dysfunction by Modulating SIRT1 in Endothelial Cells. *Molecular Nutrition & Food Research, 62*(11), e1700928. https://doi.org/10.1002/mnfr.201700928

Wang, Y., Liang, Y., & Vanhoutte, P. M. (2011). SIRT1 and AMPK in regulating mammalian senescence : A critical review and a working model. *FEBS Letters, 585*(7), 986–994. https://doi.org/10.1016/j.febslet.2010.11.047

Willems, M. E. T., Şahin, M. A., & Cook, M. D. (2018).
Matcha Green Tea Drinks Enhance Fat Oxidation
During Brisk Walking in Females. *International
Journal of Sport Nutrition and Exercise Metabolism,
28*(5), 536–541. https://doi.org/10.1123/ijsnem.2017-
0237

Yan, Z., Zhang, X., Li, C., Jiao, S., & Dong, W. (2017).
Association between consumption of soy and risk of
cardiovascular disease: A meta-analysis of
observational studies. *European Journal of Preventive
Cardiology, 24*(7), 735–747.
https://doi.org/10.1177/2047487316686441

Yang, J., Mao, Q.-X., Xu, H.-X., Ma, X., & Zeng, C.-Y.
(2014). Tea consumption and risk of type 2 diabetes
mellitus: a systematic review and meta-analysis
update. *BMJ Open, 4*(7), e005632.
https://doi.org/10.1136/bmjopen-2014-005632

Zheng, J., Zheng, S., Feng, Q., Zhang, Q., & Xiao, X.
(2017). Dietary capsaicin and its anti-obesity potency:
from mechanism to clinical implications. *Bioscience
Reports, 37*(3).
https://doi.org/10.1042/BSR20170286